Current Controversies in Maxillofacial Trauma

Guest Editors

DANIEL M. LASKIN, DDS, MS
A. OMAR ABUBAKER, DMD, PhD

ORAL AND MAXILLOFACIAL SURGERY CLINICS OF NORTH AMERICA

www.oralmaxsurgery.theclinics.com

Consulting Editor
RICHARD H. HAUG, DDS

May 2009 • Volume 21 • Number 2

SAUNDERS an imprint of ELSEVIER, Inc.

W.B. SAUNDERS COMPANY
A Division of Elsevier Inc.

1600 John F. Kennedy Blvd. • Suite 1800 • Philadelphia, PA 19103-2899

www.oralmaxsurgery.theclinics.com

ORAL AND MAXILLOFACIAL SURGERY CLINICS OF NORTH AMERICA Volume 21, Number 2
May 2009 ISSN 1042-3699, ISBN-13: 978-1-4377-0513-3, ISBN-10: 1-4377-0513-8

Editor: John Vassallo; j.vassallo@elsevier.com
Developmental Editor: Theresa Collier

Oral and Maxillofacial Surgery Clinics of North America (ISSN 1042-3699) is published quarterly by Elsevier Inc., 360 Park Avenue South, New York, NY 10010-1710. Months of issue are February, May, August, and November. Business and Editorial Offices: 1600 John F. Kennedy Blvd., Suite 1800, Philadelphia, PA 19103-2899. Periodicals postage paid at New York, NY and additional mailing offices. Subscription prices are $271.00 per year for US individuals, $401.00 per year for US institutions, $125.00 per year for US students and residents, $313.00 per year for Canadian individuals, $478.00 per year for Canadian institutions, $362.00 per year for international individuals, $478.00 per year for international institutions and $170.00 per year for Canadian and foreign students/residents. To receive student/resident rate, orders must be accompanied by name or affiliated institution, date of term, and the *signature* of program/residency coordinator on institution letterhead. Orders will be billed at individual rate until proof of status is received. Foreign air speed delivery is included in all *Clinics* subscription prices. All prices are subject to change without notice. **POSTMASTER:** Send address changes to *Oral and Maxillofacial Surgery Clinics of North America,* Elsevier Periodicals Customer Service, 11830 Westline Industrial Drive, St. Louis, MO 63146. Tel: 1-800-654-2452 (U.S. and Canada); 314-453-7041 (outside U.S. and Canada). Fax: 314-523-5170. E-mail: journalscustomerservice-usa@elsevier.com (for print support); journalsonlinesupport-usa@elsevier.com (for online support).

Reprints. For copies of 100 or more, of articles in this publication, please contact the Commercial Reprints Department, Elsevier Inc., 360 Park Avenue South, New York, NY 10010-1710. Tel.: 212-633-3812; Fax: 212-462-1935; Email: reprints@elsevier.com.

Oral and Maxillofacial Surgery Clinics of North America is covered in MEDLINE/PubMed (*Index Medicus*).

Printed and bound by CPI Group (UK) Ltd, Croydon, CR0 4YY

Transferred to Digital Print 2011

Contributors

CONSULTING EDITOR

RICHARD H. HAUG, DDS
Provost's Distinguished Service Professor,
University of Kentucky College of Dentistry,
Chandler Medical Center, Lexington, Kentucky

GUEST EDITORS

DANIEL M. LASKIN, DDS, MS
Professor and Chairman Emeritus, Department
of Oral and Maxillofacial Surgery, Virginia
Commonwealth University School of Dentistry
and Virginia Commonwealth University
Medical Center, Richmond, Virginia

A. OMAR ABUBAKER, DMD, PhD
Professor and Chairman, Department of Oral
and Maxillofacial Surgery, Virginia
Commonwealth University School of Dentistry
and Virginia Commonwealth University
Medical Center, Richmond, Virginia

AUTHORS

A. OMAR ABUBAKER, DMD, PhD
Professor and Chairman, Department of Oral
and Maxillofacial Surgery, Virginia
Commonwealth University School of Dentistry
and Virginia Commonwealth University
Medical Center, Richmond, Virginia

ERON ALDRIDGE, MD
Dental Student, University of Kentucky College
of Dentistry, Chandler Medical Center,
Lexington, Kentucky

BRIAN ALPERT, DDS
Chairman and Professor of Oral & Maxillofacial
Surgery, University of Louisville School of
Dentistry; and Chief, OMFS and Dentistry,
University of Louisville Hospital, Kentucky;
Louisville, Kentucky

R. BRYAN BELL, DDS, MD, FACS
Attending Head and Neck Surgeon and Director
of Resident Education, Oral and Maxillofacial
Surgery Service, Legacy Emanuel Hospital and
Health Center; Clinical Associate Professor,
Oregon Health & Science University, Portland,
Oregon; and Adjunct Assistant Professor,
University of Washington, Seattle,
Washington

HANI BRAIDY, DMD
Assistant Professor, Department of Oral and
Maxillofacial Surgery, University of Medicine and
Dentistry of New Jersey, Newark, New Jersey

BRYAN S. CHRISTENSEN, DMD
Resident, Oral and Maxillofacial Surgery,
University of Oklahoma, Oklahoma City,
Oklahoma

EDWARD ELLIS III, DDS, MS
Professor of Oral and Maxillofacial Surgery,
University of Texas Southwestern Medical
Center, Dallas, Texas

RICHARD H. HAUG, DDS
Provost's Distinguished Service Professor,
University of Kentucky College of Dentistry,
Chandler Medical Center, Lexington, Kentucky

RISTO KONTIO, MD, DDS, PhD
Senior Maxillofacial Surgeon, Department of
Oral and Maxillofacial Surgery, Helsinki
University Central Hospital, Helsinki, Finland

GEORGE M. KUSHNER, DMD, MD
Professor and Director, Advanced Education
Program in Oral & Maxillofacial Surgery,
University of Louisville School of Dentistry,
Louisville, Kentucky

DANIEL M. LASKIN, DDS, MS
Professor and Chairman Emeritus, Department of Oral and Maxillofacial Surgery, Virginia Commonwealth University School of Dentistry and Virginia Commonwealth University Medical Center, Richmond, Virginia

CHRISTIAN LINDQVIST, MD, DDS, PhD
Professor and Chair, Department of Oral and Maxillofacial Surgery, Helsinki University Central Hospital; and Institute of Dentistry, University of Helsinki, Helsinki, Finland

MATTHEW J. MADSEN, DMD
Resident, Department of Oral and Maxillofacial Surgery, University of Louisville School of Dentistry, Louisville, Kentucky

ROBERT W.T. MYALL, BDS, MD, FDS, FRCD(C)
Professor of Oral & Maxillofacial Surgery, School of Dentistry, Oregon Health & Science University; and Professor of Surgery, School of Medicine, Oregon Health & Science University, Portland, Oregon

HARRY PAPADOPOULOS, DDS, MD
Clinical Associate Professor, Division of Oral & Maxillofacial Surgery, Department of Oral Surgery & Hospital Dentistry, Indiana

University; and Director, Oral & Maxillofacial Surgery Residency Training Program, Indiana University, Indianapolis, Indiana

NADER K. SALIB, DDS
Third Year Resident, Division of Oral & Maxillofacial Surgery, Department of Oral Surgery & Hospital Dentistry, Indiana University, Indianapolis, Indiana

PANAGIOTIS K. STEFANOPOULOS, DDS, MAJ (DC)
Hellenic Army, Oral and Maxillofacial Surgery Department, Athens, Greece

PAUL S. TIWANA, DDS, MD, MS
Assistant Professor of Oral and Maxillofacial Surgery, University of Louisville School of Dentistry; and Chief, Pediatric OMFS, Kosair-Children's Hospital, Louisville, Kentucky

JOSEPH E. VAN SICKELS, DDS
Professor and Chief, Division of Oral and Maxillofacial Surgery, University of Kentucky, Lexington, Kentucky

VINCENT B. ZICCARDI, DDS, MD
Associate Professor and Chair, Department of Oral and Maxillofacial Surgery, University of Medicine and Dentistry of New Jersey, Surgery, Newark, New Jersey

Contents

follow-up. In the adult, it is important to restore ramus height by an open reduction when (1) there are bilateral fractures without contact of the segments, (2) there is a unilateral fracture in an edentulous patient, or (3) there is a unilateral fracture in a dentulous patient with an unstable occlusion. Open reduction is also necessary when there is a need to establish a stable mandibular base for the treatment of associated midface fractures or when there is mechanical interference with establishing a proper occlusion.

Management of Mandibular Fractures in Children   197

Robert W.T. Myall

To guide surgeons treating mandibular fractures in children, this article first reviews the growth of the mandible, describes how injury can affect such growth, and explains how to harness the process of growth to good effect. This information is important in making therapeutic decisions about the management of such injuries. The article then reviews the various opinions regarding diagnosis, treatment, and outcomes. Then, as a counterpoint, the author presents his own approach developed over 30 years as a pediatric oral and maxillofacial surgeon.

Management of Nasal Fractures   203

Vincent B. Ziccardi and Hani Braidy

The goal of treatment for nasal fractures is to restore the pretraumatic state and normal function. The decision by the surgeon regarding the surgical approach should be based on the degree of injury, the presence of concomitant facial injuries, patient compliance, training of the surgeon, and the presence and degree of septal injury. The use of a closed or open approach will then depend on the extent of the injury.

Management of Orbital Fractures   209

Risto Kontio and Christian Lindqvist

Trauma to the orbit is always complex, and adequate therapy requires that the surgeon be familiar with the detailed anatomy of the orbit and the pattern of injury of the soft and hard tissue components. Preoperative CT, MRI scans, or both are mandatory for diagnosis and proper planning of reconstruction. Although several autogenous and alloplastic materials are available, autogenous bone grafting seems to give the best results. Resorbable materials cannot be recommended for large defects. Instead, either bone or titanium must be considered to achieve a long-lasting, accurate restoration of bony orbital anatomy and dimension. Postoperative CT scan evaluation is of utmost importance regardless of the reconstruction method used.

Management of Naso-Orbital-Ethmoidal Fractures   221

Harry Papadopoulos and Nader K. Salib

Naso-orbital-ethmoidal fractures are arguably the most challenging fractures of the facial skeleton to restore properly. This article discusses their proper diagnosis, describes some of the controversies in their management, and makes recommendations regarding their proper treatment.

Management of Frontal Sinus Fractures   227

R. Bryan Bell

The goals in the treatment of frontal sinus injuries are to provide an esthetic outcome, restore function, and prevent complications. However, there is no consensus as to how to best achieve these goals. Unfortunately, the questions that Stanley proposed in 1989 still lack definitive answers more than 19 years later: (1) Which fractures, if left untreated, will lead to an immediate or delayed complication? and (2) What is the appropriate surgical procedure if treatment of the fracture is deemed necessary? This article discusses the controversies in the surgical treatment of such fractures and provides a scientific rationale for proper management.

Surgical repair of injuries to the parotid gland and its duct have been described in the literature for more than 100 years. Injury to the glandular structures are usually associated with penetrating wounds of the face and often involve concomitant damage to adjacent structures, including the facial nerve, the ear, and the nearby bony structures. Most investigators agree that management of these injuries depends on the location of the damage. However, there are differences of opinion as to the proper management of the repair when the injury to the glandular system is discovered early or late.

Bite wounds are especially prone to infectious complications, both local and systemic. In bite wounds to the face, such complications can create more difficulties than the initial tissue damage itself for the task of restoring an esthetic appearance. Management should aim to neutralize this potential for infection and provide an infection-free environment for wound healing. Wound cleansing followed by primary closure is the treatment of choice, and the use of prophylactic antibiotics may further decrease the risk of infection. Delay in presentation beyond 24 hours is not necessarily a contraindication to immediate repair, but excessive crushing of the tissues or extensive edema usually dictates a more conservative approach, such as delayed closure.

In managing traumatic wounds, the primary goal is to achieve rapid healing with optimal functional and esthetic results. This is best accomplished by providing an environment that prevents infection of the wound during healing. Despite good wound care, some infections still occur. Accordingly, some investigators argue that prophylactic antibiotics have an important role in the management of certain types of wounds. This article reviews the basis of antibiotic use in preventing wound infection in general and its use in oral and facial wounds in particular.

Oral and Maxillofacial Surgery Clinics of North America

THE CLINICS ARE NOW AVAILABLE ONLINE!

Access your subscription at:
www.theclinics.com

Preface

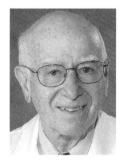 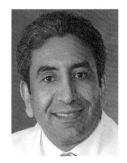

Daniel M. Laskin, DDS, MS   A. Omar Abubaker, DMD, PhD
Guest Editors

Controversy can be defined as a dispute, generally with a right and a wrong side of the argument. Controversy can also be defined as a discussion marked by the expression of opposing views. The articles in this issue best fit this definition because, when there are different approaches to surgical management, it is often not a matter of right or wrong, but rather what the surgeon believes gives the best results. It is regrettable that in the treatment of many kinds of traumatic injuries of the maxillofacial region, too few randomized, controlled studies are available to supply strong supporting evidence for definitely selecting one surgical technique or procedure over another. Therefore, we have to rely upon expert opinion, as well as the literature, to guide us in the decision-making process.

For this issue, we are fortunate to have recruited many experienced national and international oral and maxillofacial surgeons as authors. In preparing their contributions, they were asked to present the evidence from the literature on each side of an issue and to then suggest the method of treatment that, in their opinion, they considered most likely to provide the best outcomes. They are

to be congratulated on admirably fulfilling this task and we thank them for their efforts.

It is unfortunate that there are still so many controversial areas in the management of maxillofacial trauma. In this issue, we have chosen to address those involving situations most frequently encountered by the oral and maxillofacial surgeon. It is our hope that the information provided will either confirm those opinions that you now hold, or convince you to change when there appears to be a strong argument for doing so. Ultimately, the goal is to help provide the best care for our patients.

Daniel M. Laskin, DDS, MS
A. Omar Abubaker, DMD, PhD

Department of Oral and Maxillofacial Surgery
VCU School of Dentistry and VCU Medical Center
521 North 11th Street
PO Box 980566
Richmond, VA 23298-0566, USA

E-mail addresses:
dmlaskin@vcu.edu (D.M. Laskin)
omar_abubaker@vcu.edu (A.O. Abubaker)

doi:10.1016/j.coms.2009.01.001

Management of Fractures Through the Angle of the Mandible

Edward Ellis III, DDS, MS

KEYWORDS

• Mandibular fracture • Angle fracture • Miniplate

Fracture through the angle of the mandible is one of the most common maxillofacial injuries sustained in modern societies. Among issues related to the treatment of maxillofacial injuries, those concerning angle fractures are the most hotly debated, with the exception perhaps of those concerning the condylar process of the mandible. There are several reasons for this controversy about treatment of angle fractures, a controversy too often made up of arguments founded on emotion rather than on scientific information. This article discusses some of the controversies in the management of such fractures.

DEFINITION

There is no consensus in the literature about the definition of an "angle" fracture of the mandible. However, there are two points of agreement. The first is that the term *angle* refers to an anatomic region, although some disagree about what encompasses that region. The second point of agreement is the position where the fracture is located on the superior aspect of the mandible: The fracture line starts in the area where the anterior border of the mandibular ramus meets the body of the mandible, usually in the region where the third molar is or was. If the third molar is present, it may be located anywhere along the root of this tooth. Sometimes the fracture may be along the distal root, with the tooth remaining within the distal segment of the mandible. Other times, the fracture is located along the mesial root, with the tooth remaining within the proximal segment. Still other times, the fracture runs through the middle of the tooth with the tooth lying

almost free within the fracture, especially if the roots are incompletely formed and the tooth is unerupted. Occasionally, the fracture will also split the tooth, with one root remaining in the proximal and one in the distal segment (**Fig. 1**). When the tooth is fractured, it is almost always an erupted tooth. When the third molar is missing, the fracture is usually along the distal root of the second molar, exposing the root to the fracture. However, the fracture may be further posterior to the second molar, occurring in the area where the third molar would normally be, leaving a layer of bone covering the roots of the second molar.

The greatest disagreement regarding the angle fracture is its location on the inferior or posterior mandibular border. Does the "angle" fracture have to extend through the gonial angle of the mandible? Most of the literature indicates that the fracture extends to the inferior border anterior to the gonial angle. However, in the author's experience, the vast majority of fractures of the angle of the mandible extend vertically from the region of the third molar inferiorly through the inferior border of the mandible (see **Fig. 1**). They can, however, extend posteriorly as they pass inferiorly. In a small percentage of cases (approximately 8%), the fracture extends toward the gonial angle of the mandible (**Fig. 2**), and occasionally even slightly above it (**Fig. 3**). In extremely rare cases, the fracture can extend anteriorly, exiting the inferior border in a location that is anterior to the region where it occurred along the superior border.

Biomechanically, any fracture that extends from the third molar region to the inferior or posterior border is similar in that the muscles that elevate the mandible tend to cause the ramus to rotate

Oral and Maxillofacial Surgery, University of Texas Southwestern Medical Center, 5323 Harry Hines Blvd., Dallas, TX 75390-9109, USA
E-mail address: edward.ellis@utsouthwestern.edu

Oral Maxillofacial Surg Clin N Am 21 (2009) 163–174
doi:10.1016/j.coms.2008.12.004
1042-3699/08/$ – see front matter © 2009 Elsevier Inc. All rights reserved.

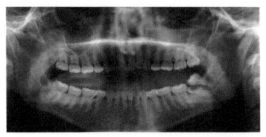

Fig. 1. Panoramic radiograph of a fracture through the mandibular angle and also through the third molar. The location of this fracture could be considered typical in that it extends from the third molar area inferiorly, exiting through the inferior border of the mandible.

anterosuperiorly. Thus a fracture of the mandibular "angle" can be variable in its course through the mandible (**Fig. 4**).

ANGLE FRACTURE CHARACTERISTICS

With any fracture there are certain characteristics that provide useful information on the "nature" or the "character" of the injury. Six descriptors are commonly used, the first being location, which in this case is the angle region of the mandible. The others are whether the fracture is:

- Complete or incomplete (**Fig. 5**)
- Linear (or simple) (see **Figs. 1–3** and **5**) or comminuted (**Fig. 6**)
- Compound or closed (ie, noncompound) (see **Figs. 1–3**)
- Displaced or nondisplaced (**Fig. 7**A)
- Mobile or nonmobile

Much of the controversy regarding management of angle fractures relates to the inclusion of different types of angle fractures in the same series without distinguishing among them.

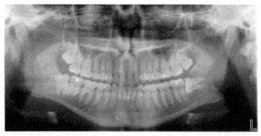

Fig. 2. Panoramic radiograph of a fracture extending from the third molar area through the gonial angle of the mandible.

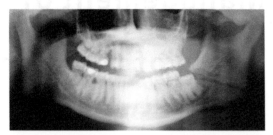

Fig. 3. Panoramic radiograph of a fracture extending from the third molar area through the posterior border of the mandibular ramus, just above the gonial angle.

ANATOMY/BIOMECHANICS

In making decisions regarding the management of angle fractures, it is important to understand the factors that account for displacement and how these can be effectively counteracted. The region of the mandibular angle is bounded by the strong elevator muscles (temporalis, masseter, medial pterygoid) that allow the generation of significant bite forces (300–400 N).[1,2] This force is significantly reduced for several weeks after a fracture of the mandible,[1,2] probably by the central nervous system inhibiting full contraction when it perceives an injury from the mechanoreceptors in the bone and soft tissues around the fracture. Fortunately, this means that fixation schemes applied to a fractured mandibular angle do not have to resist normal forces, but only have to counter the reduced forces that patients with fractures can generate.

However, even reduced contraction of the elevator muscles allows the ramus to rotate upward and forward when a fracture exists through the angle, displacing the bone fragments, especially at the superior surface (see **Fig. 7**A).

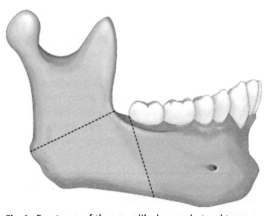

Fig. 4. Fractures of the mandibular angle tend to occur in the area between the dotted lines.

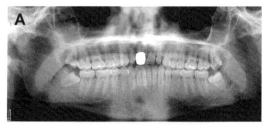

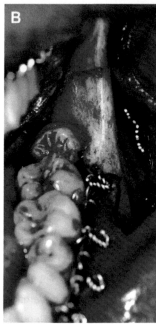

Fig. 5. (A) Panoramic radiograph of an incomplete fracture. The fracture line extends from the third molar through the inferior border of the mandible. This fracture was clinically nonmobile. (B) Exposure of the fracture shows no fracture of the buccal cortex. Presumably, the fracture line on the radiograph was through the lingual cortex or tension side of the impacted mandibular angle.

Making this movement even more likely is the action of the mandibular depressor muscles (anterior digastric, geniohyoid) that displace the anterior mandible inferiorly and posteriorly when a fracture exists posteriorly (ie, through the angle). This is why historically the angle fracture frequently required some form of fixation (eg, intraosseous wire, external pin) in addition to maxillomandibular fixation (MMF) to control the position of the ramus. Today, internal fixation devices (ie, plates, screws) are used for the same reason and to obviate postoperative MMF.

Clinical observations and biomechanical investigations have shown that during normal jaw function, tension occurs at the level of the dentition, whereas compression occurs along the lower border of the mandible.[3,4] Biomechanical investigations have also shown with simulated fractures

through the mandibular angle that the fragments separate most at the superior surface (tension zone) (**Fig. 8**). Fixation devices applied directly across the fragments are mechanically most advantageous when placed in the area where the fragments tend to separate under the influence of muscle function[5] (ie, the superior border of the mandible).

Sophisticated biomechanical models of the mandible under function have also shown that the zones of tension and compression in a mandibular angle fracture can change with different biting positions (ie, ipsilateral molar versus incisor). Thus, various fixation schemes have been developed to help "neutralize" the forces acting across a fractured mandibular angle. As is discussed below, these schemes seem completely dichotomous, probably because of our lack of a complete understanding of the masticatory system and how it responds to injury.[6]

TREATMENT

The literature is filled with dozens of studies concerning treatment of fractures through the mandibular angle. Many of them are contradictory and often the clinical results nonintuitive. However, the studies have identified some consistencies and peculiarities of angle fractures that should be discussed.

Antibiotics

Antibiotics for compound fractures of the mandibular angle should be instituted as soon after injury as possible to help prevent infection.[7,8] They should be continued at least until after surgical treatment has been provided. The "worth" of postoperative antibiotics has not been demonstrated.[9,10]

Timing of Treatment

In general, compound fractures of the mandible should be treated as soon as possible. Champy and colleagues[3] and Cawood[11] recommended that, to minimize the incidence of dehiscence and infection, miniplate osteosynthesis must be performed soon after injury. Champy and colleagues[3] recommended fixation, with no preoperative antibiotics, within 12 hours of injury. Cawood[11] extended this period to 24 hours after injury. Often, however, patients do not present for treatment until days after their injury and even when they do present early, it is not always possible to perform immediate surgery for a host of logistical reasons. Fortunately, a delay is unlikely to cause problems. No one has yet

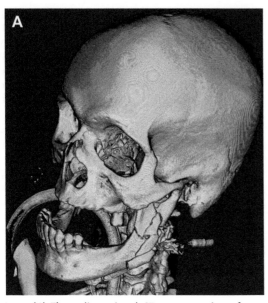

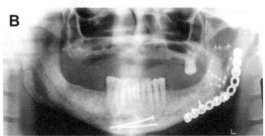

Fig. 6. (*A*) Three-dimensional CT reconstruction of a comminuted fracture through the mandibular angle. This fracture required load-bearing fixation in the form of a reconstruction bone plate (*B*). The smaller plates were used simply to maintain the position of the smaller fragments.

demonstrated a relationship between postoperative complication and the time between injury and treatment.[12-17] It seems reasonable to manage a compound fracture of the mandibular angle as soon as possible, but there is no evidence that they should be treated as emergencies.

Teeth in Line of Fracture

Third molars are commonly associated with the line of fracture through the mandibular angle. In a study of 402 angle fractures by Ellis,[18] 85% contained a third molar. Unfortunately, there is confusing information in the literature concerning the question of what to do with the tooth in the line of a mandibular angle fracture.[16,18–25]

Spiessl[19] lists three undesirable effects of extracting an *unerupted* tooth in the line of an angle fracture:

- The possibility of converting a closed fracture to an open one
- Loss of the bony buttress on the tension side (superior surface)
- Loss of the possibility for inserting a tension band plate

However, the first possibility assumes that one will treat the fracture through a transfacial approach. For those who treat fractures of the angle of the mandible through a transoral approach, the question of conversion to an open

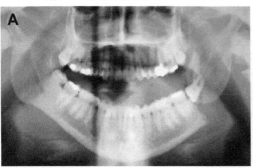

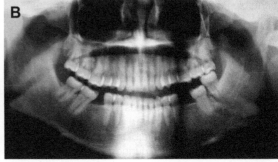

Fig. 7. Panoramic radiographs of two fractures through the mandibular angle. In the first (*A*), there is no erupted tooth in the proximal fragment to prevent upward and forward rotation of the mandibular ramus secondary to the action of the elevator muscles. In the second (*B*), an erupted third molar prevents upward and forward rotation from occurring.

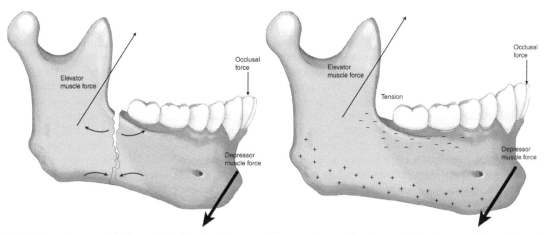

Fig. 8. When the mandibular angle is fractured, a gap at the superior surface is created by the opposing action of the elevator muscles, which rotate the mandibular ramus upwards and forward, and the depressor muscles that rotate the anterior mandible inferiorly. Thus, the superior surface of the mandible undergoes "tension," or separation. The inferior border of the mandible at the area of the fracture may stay apposed because the muscle action causes the fragments in that location to be compressed toward one another (ie, the inferior border is a zone of compression).

fracture is moot because the fracture will be opened to the oral cavity anyway during surgery. The second and third considerations assume that one will be removing bone during the extraction process, which is not usually necessary.

Spiessl[19] also recommends extraction of an *erupted* third molar when the apex is "open" to the fracture, the root is fractured, or the third molar is partially erupted.

Some data in the literature address this issue. When open reduction and internal fixation is selected as the treatment, there seems to be some agreement that the presence of a third molar associated with a fracture through the angle of the mandible increases the risk of infection irrespective of whether or not the tooth is erupted or impacted, or whether or not the tooth is removed during surgery.[18,25] For closed treatment, there seems to be no difference in the rate of infection irrespective of whether the tooth was removed or left in place.[22,24] With literature providing no clear guidance, clinicians must use their best judgment in weighing the benefits and risks of removing a third molar in the line of an angle fracture against the benefits and risks of leaving it.

Closed Versus Open Reduction (and Internal Fixation)

In the preantibiotic era, most fractures of the mandible were treated closed, using MMF, splints, and similar devices. During that period, fractures through the mandibular angle were those most likely to undergo open reduction and internal fixation because, in most cases of angle fracture, the mandibular ramus, to which the powerful elevator

muscles are attached, could not be controlled by MMF. Rotation of the ramus upwards and forward often occurred, resulting in nonunion, malunion, intraoral exposure of the rotated ramus, and similar problems. External pin fixation and a host of "gadgets" were therefore employed to prevent displacement of the fragments. Thus, closed treatment for angle fractures using MMF has limited application unless there is an erupted tooth in the proximal segment that can provide a vertical "stop" to prevent rotation of the ramus (**Fig. 7**B).

Most fractures of the mandibular angle are treated by open reduction and internal fixation. Even when the fracture is not displaced, open treatment is usually provided so that internal fixation devices can be placed to maintain the alignment of the fragments and obviate postoperative MMF.

Internal Fixation Schemes

Every type of internal fixation device, from wire to reconstruction bone plate, has been used to provide stability across the fractured angle of the mandible. When wire fixation is applied, postoperative MMF is required for at least 4 to 5 weeks to immobilize the fractured fragments and allow osseous union to commence.[26]

All other forms of internal fixation devices obviate postoperative MMF. However, they vary widely in the amount of stability they provide to the fractured fragments. Most of the confusion and debate about the most appropriate treatment of fractures of the mandibular angle arises from the great difference in stability of the various devices.

There are two general philosophies espoused by users of plate and screw fixation for mandibular fractures. One group feels that plate and screw fixation should provide sufficient rigidity to the fragments to prevent interfragmentary mobility during active use of the mandible. This group recommends placing large bone plates fastened with bicortical bone screws, one large and one small bone plate, or two small plates to provide such rigidity.[19,27–33] For these surgeons, the goal of treatment of mandibular fractures is primary bone union, which necessitates absolute immobility of fragments.

In 1973, Michelet[34] reported on the treatment of mandibular fractures using small, easily bendable noncompression bone plates, placed transorally and attached with monocortical screws. Champy and colleagues[3] performed several investigations with a "miniplate" system to validate the technique. In their experiments, they determined the "ideal lines of osteosynthesis" in the mandible, or the locations where bone plate fixation should provide the most stable means of fixation. For fractures of the mandibular angle, the most effective plate location was found to be along the superior border of the mandible (**Fig. 9**). Because the bone plates were small and the screws monocortical, fixation could be applied in these most mechanically advantageous areas without damaging teeth. For surgeons using this approach, absolute immobilization of bone fragments and primary bone union was deemed unnecessary. Clinical studies since have proven the usefulness of this technique.[11,17,35–42]

It has been a generally accepted theorem that more stability between the fractured bone fragments provides a better environment for bone healing. However, there seems to be an inconsistency between the results of biomechanical models of fixation devices applied to simulated fractures of the mandibular angle and clinical outcomes. All biomechanical models developed to date have shown that two points of fixation (ie, two bone plates) provide much more stability than does one.[4,30,31,43,44] Also, several biomechanical studies have shown that three-dimensional "strut" plates (**Fig. 10**) provide more stability than one miniplate.[44–49] These models have also shown that a single miniplate cannot control bending or torsional forces, especially when the mandible is loaded ipsilaterally. Based upon such biomechanical studies, some investigators have advocated the use of two miniplates for fractures of the mandibular angle rather than one.[29–32,50,51]

Unfortunately, clinical results are variable concerning the amount of stability that must be provided across the fractured angle of the mandible. Fox and Kellman[32] and others[29,51] have found advantages to the routine use of two plates rather than one. However, other clinical results do not corroborate these clinical results and more elaborate biomechanical tests have failed to show the benefit of a second miniplate. Ellis and Walker[15] found in their patient population a very high rate of major complications (29%), mostly infections, when angle fractures were treated with two miniplates. In fact, the use of a single miniplate, as

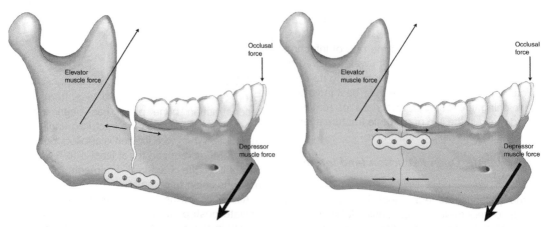

Fig. 9. For fractures of the angle, a plate applied at the superior border of the mandible is much more effective than a plate applied at the inferior border. This is because metallic plates have good tensile strength. When even small plates are applied to the area that tends to separate under function (zone of tension), the plate prevents separation. When a plate is located in the area of the fracture that does not tend to separate under function (zone of compression), the plate is stressed in line, and small plates will bend, creating an unstable osteosynthesis.

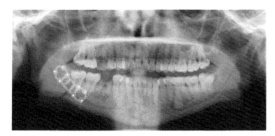

Fig. 10. Panoramic radiograph showing the use of a three-dimensional "strut" or "geometic" plate applied to a fractured mandibular angle.

advocated by Champy,[3] was found to be very successful in their patient population.[17] Similarly, clinical studies by Shierle and collegues[52] and Siddiqui and collegues[53] found that two-plate fixation does not offer advantages over single-plate fixation in general when treating fractures through the angle of the mandible. The results of such studies indicate that biomechanics are only one factor to be considered when treating fractures. Many others may be more important. Perhaps improved maintenance of the blood supply to the bone because of limited dissection is one such factor.[54–56] Rudderman and colleagues[6] have also offered biomechanical explanations for the success of a single miniplate used to treat fractures of the mandibular angle. They feel that forces are not only distributed through the bones and fixation devices, but also through the soft tissues, creating circuits of force. Such a model explains why a single miniplate can be very successful in the management of fracture through the angle of the mandible. A study in 2005 by Gear and colleagues[57] has shown that the most commonly used method of stabilizing fractures through the angle of the mandible by AO/ASIF (Arbeitsgemeinschaft für Osteosynthesefragen–Association for the Study of Internal Fixation) surgeons in North America and Europe is with a single miniplate.

However, it is clear that a single miniplate cannot always provide sufficient stability to a fractured mandibular angle. There are two general situations in which more fixation is required. The first is the comminuted fracture through the angle of the mandible. This requires load-bearing fixation that can only be provided using a reconstruction bone plate that is secured with at least three screws on each side and that spans the area of the comminution (**Fig. 6**). For purposes of this article, I did not deal with comminuted or defect fractures and instead discussed the treatment of the more common fracture through the angle of the mandible: the complete, linear, displaced, mobile, compound fracture that is almost always the result of interpersonal violence.

The second and more common situation where one would need more stability across the fractured mandibular angle is when there is an associated fracture elsewhere in the mandible that will either be treated closed or treated with nonrigid fixation. For example, the combination of a fracture through the angle and the contralateral condylar process creates a biomechanical environment that is much more complex than an isolated fracture of the mandible. If one chooses to treat the condylar process fracture closed using functional therapy (no MMF), one should place rigid fixation on the fracture through the mandibular angle to prevent torsional forces from displacing the inferior border of the mandible in the area of the angle fracture. A second miniplate applied further inferiorly than the first provides rigid fixation of the angle fracture. One could also use a more rigid plate, or one of the "geometric" strut or three-dimensional bone plates (**Fig. 10**), to provide rigid fixation of the fractured angle. If, on the other hand, one chooses to perform open reduction and internal fixation of the condylar process fracture, one could then treat the mandibular angle fracture as an "isolated" fracture, with a single miniplate.

The most common situation is the combination of fractures through both the mandibular angle and the contralateral body or symphysis. The biomechanics of this fracture pattern are much more complicated than those associated with an isolated fracture of either region. One of the two fractures must be made rigid (ie, no micromotion possible), and then the other can be treated with a single miniplate. In practice, the simplest way to manage this combination of fractures is to apply rigid fixation to the most accessible fracture (ie, the symphysis or body fracture) and then the angle fracture can be treated as an "isolated" fracture with a single miniplate. Rigid fixation of the body or symphysis fracture can be performed with a thicker, stronger plate; two miniplates; lag screws; or a combination of these (**Fig. 11**).

POSTOPERATIVE CARE

After surgery for fractures through the mandibular angle, patients are managed similarly to those with fractures in other parts of the mandible. Postsurgical training elastics should only be used if the occlusion is not perfect a day or so after surgery. There is no evidence that maintaining patients on antibiotics after surgery is of any benefit.[9,10] Routine use of a chlorhexidine mouth rinse makes good sense, as does the use of good oral hygiene measures.

Postoperative radiographs taken within a few days postoperatively may sometimes reveal

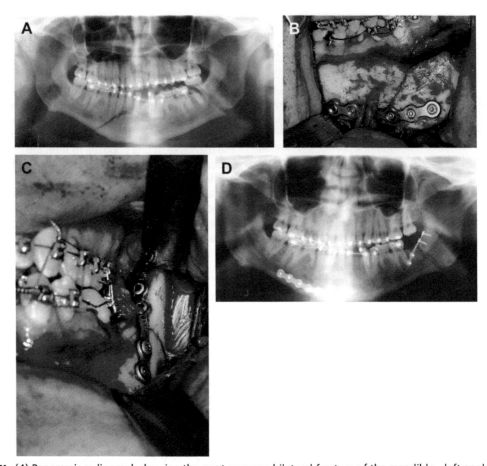

Fig. 11. (*A*) Panoramic radiograph showing the most common bilateral fracture of the mandible—left angle plus right body/symphysis. The fracture of the right body/symphysis was treated with "rigid" fixation, using a bone plate that is much thicker and stronger than a miniplate (*B*). The fractured angle was then treated using a standard malleable miniplate (*C*). Postoperative radiograph (*D*) shows the reduction.

a 2- to 4-mm gap at the inferior border (**Fig. 12**A). The appearance of this gap raises the issue of whether the patient should then be placed into MMF. Surprisingly, this gap rarely causes a malocclusion. When there is a malocclusion, it is usually a slight posterior open-bite on the side of the angle fracture. In such cases, light vertical elastics can be used to settle the teeth into occlusion. When a single miniplate is used, the inferior border gap slowly disappears in subsequent weeks because of the biomechanics of function, whereby the elevator muscles rotate the ramus anteriorly and superiorly, with the superior border plate as the fulcrum, and close the gap (**Fig. 12**B). When there is a gap at the inferior border in a patient

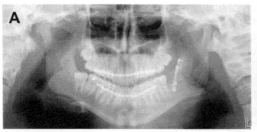
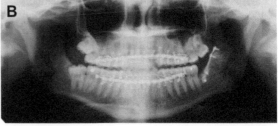

Fig. 12. (*A*) Immediate postoperative panoramic radiograph showing a gap in the fracture line at the inferior border. (*B*) Another radiograph taken a few weeks later shows that the gap has closed.

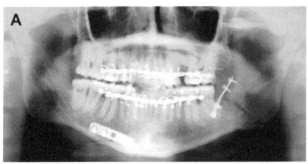
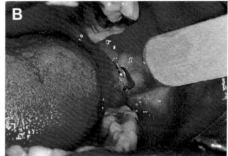

Fig. 13. (*A*) Panoramic radiograph showing loosening of the posterior screws. (*B*) Exposure of the bone plate through the mucosa.

with two miniplates attached to the mandible, the gap cannot close on its own, but will fill with new bone over time.

COMPLICATIONS

The management of mandibular angle fractures has traditionally been associated with a high postoperative complication rate (up to 33%).[15,17,33,38,58–67] These can be divided into intraoperative and postoperative complications. Intraoperative complications are rare. The main intraoperative hazard is injury to the inferior alveolar neurovascular bundle. The anterior screws are often located right over the inferior alveolar canal and those used are frequently too long. However, with careful drilling through only the outer cortex and use of 5- or 6-mm screws, which are sufficient, injury to the contents of the canal can be avoided.

Fractures through the angle of the mandible are associated with a high incidence of postoperative complications. These can be broken down into minor and major complications. Minor complications are those that are amenable to treatment in the outpatient clinic. The incidence of reported

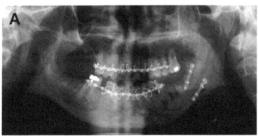

Fig. 14. (*A*) Panoramic radiograph showing loss of bone around the screws and loosening of screws. (*B*) Intraoperative photograph showing loose superior border bone and devitalization and resorption of the buccal plate. (*C*) Intraoperative photograph showing loose screws and resorption of buccal plate of bone. In this case, the fracture was united by healing of the lingual cortex.

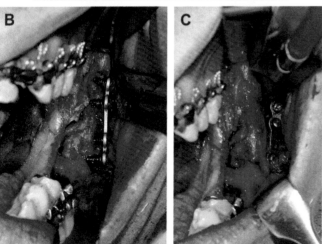

minor complications varies widely in the literature, but constituted the majority of total complications (85%) in a study by Walker and Ellis[17] when a single miniplate was used. Minor complications are minor infections, swelling without discharge of pus, or complaints of pain in the area of the bone plate. In most patients with minor complications, the fractures heal uneventfully with simple treatment, such as oral antibiotics and wound care. Loosening of the screws (**Fig. 13**A) and exposure of the superior border bone plate through the gingiva (**Fig. 13**B), with or without swelling or mild infection, is uncommon. When it occurs, the plate does not have to be removed immediately. Rather, the problem can be easily treated by placing the patient on antibiotics and a chlorhexadine rinse until healing occurs. Then the plate can be removed under local anesthesia in the clinic.

Major complications are uncommon when a single miniplate is used for treatment of fractures through the mandibular angle. The most common major complications are infections requiring extraoral incision and drainage, intravenous antibiotics, debridement of nonvital bone, and removal of the bone plate. However, on occasion, and especially after an infection, the result is a fibrous union that requires more stable fixation and possibly bone grafting.

Major complications are greater with the use of two rather than one miniplate.[15,17] Walker and Ellis[15] noted a significant occurrence of such complications (28%) as late dehiscence of the incision, swelling, granulation tissue formation, and the need for plate removal or debridement of nonvital bone (**Fig. 14**). Typically, the fracture had healed adequately at the time of debridement/plate removal so no additional fixation was required. However, this procedure greatly increased the cost of treatment.

SUMMARY

Fractures through the angle of the mandible will continue to be common. Treatment variables and fixation schemes will likely be investigated further in an attempt to improve treatment outcomes and simplify treatment. At present, the technique originally advocated by Champy[3] seems to the technique of choice for noncomminuted fractures of the mandibular angle that occur in isolation or when applied to the multiply-fractured mandible when the other fractures can be rigidly stabilized.

REFERENCES

1. Tate GS, Ellis E, Throckmorton GS, et al. Bite forces in patients treated for mandibular angle fractures—implications for fixation recommendations. J Oral Maxillofac Surg 1994;52:734–6.

2. Gerlach KL, Schwarz A. Bite forces in patients after treatment of mandibular angle fractures with miniplate osteosynthesis according to Champy. Int J Oral Maxillofac Surg 2002;31:345–8.

3. Champy M, Lodde JH, Must D, et al. Mandibular osteosynthesis by miniature screwed plates via buccal approach. J Maxillofac Surg 1978;6:14–9.

4. Kroon FH, Mathisson M, Cordey JR, et al. The use of miniplates in mandibular fractures. J Craniomaxillofac Surg 1991;19:199–204.

5. Pauwels F. Grundriss einer biomechanik der frakturheilung. Verh Dtsch Orthop Ges 1940;34:62–7 [German].

6. Rudderman RH, Mullen RL, Phillips JH, et al. The biophysics of mandibular fractures: an evolution toward understanding. Plast Reconstr Surg 2008; 121:596–607.

7. Zallen RD, Curry IT. A study of antibiotic usage in compound mandibular fractures. J Oral Surg 1975; 33:431–4.

8. Chole RA, Yee J. Antiotic prophylaxis for facial fractures. Arch Otolaryngol Head Neck Surg 1987;113: 1055–7.

9. Abubaker A, Rollert M. Postoperative antibiotic prophylaxis in mandibular fractures: a preliminary randomized, double-blind, and placebo-controlled clinical study. J Oral Maxillofac Surg 2001;59: 1415–9.

10. Miles BA, Potter JK, Ellis E, et al. The efficacy of postoperative antibiotic regimens in the open treatment of mandibular fractures: a prospective randomized trial. J Oral Maxillofac Surg 2006;64:576–82.

11. Cawood JI. Small plate osteosynthesis of mandibular fractures. Br J Oral Maxillofac Surg 1985;23: 77–91.

12. Tuovinen V, Norholt SE, Sindet-Pedersen S, et al. A retrospective analysis of 279 patients with isolated mandibular fractures treated with titanium miniplates. J Oral Maxillofac Surg 1994;52:931–5.

13. Barnard NA, Hook P. Delayed miniplate osteosynthesis for mandibular fractures. Br J Oral Maxillofac Surg 1991;29:357 [Letter to the Editor].

14. Smith WP. Delayed miniplate osteosynthesis for mandibular fractures. Br J Oral Maxillofac Surg 1991;29:73–6.

15. Ellis E, Walker L. Treatment of mandibular angle fractures using two noncompression miniplates. J Oral Maxillofac Surg 1994;52:1032–6.

16. Marker P, Eckerdal A, Smith-Sivertsen C, et al. Incompletely erupted third molars in the line of mandibular fractures. A retrospective analysis of 57 cases. Oral Surg 1994;78:426–31.

17. Ellis E, Walker LR. Treatment of mandibular angle fractures using one noncompression miniplate. J Oral Maxillofac Surg 1996;54:864–71.

18. Ellis E. Outcomes of patients with teeth in the line of mandibular angle fractures treated with stable internal fixation. J Oral Maxillofac Surg 2002;60: 863–5.

19. Spiessl B. Closed fractures. Chapter 5. In: Spiessl B, editor. Internal fixation of the mandible. Berlin: Springer-Verlag; 1989. p. 199.

20. Thaller SR, Mabourakh S. Teeth located in the line of mandibular fracture. J Craniofac Surg 1994;5:16–9.

21. Gerbino F, Tarello M, Fasolis PP, et al. De Gioanni: rigid fixation with teeth in the line of mandibular fractures. Int J Oral Maxillofac Surg 1997;26:182–6.

22. Rubin MM, Koll TJ, Sadoff RS, et al. Morbidity associated with incompletely erupted third molars in the line of mandibular fractures. J Oral Maxillofac Surg 1990;48:1045–7.

23. Shetty V, Freymiller E. Teeth in the line of fracture: a review. J Oral Maxillofac Surg 1989;47:1303–6.

24. Anastassov DT, Vuvakis VM. Mandibular fracture complications associated with the third molar lying in the fracture line. Folia Med (Plovdiv) 2000;42: 41–6.

25. Soriano E, Kankou V, Morand B, et al. Fractures of the mandibular angle: factors predictive of infectious complications. Rev Stomatol Chir Maxillofac 2005; 106:146–8.

26. Juniper RP, Awty MD. The immobilization period for fractures of the mandibular body. Oral Surg 1973; 36:157–63.

27. Spiessl B. New concepts in maxillofacial bone surgery. In: Spiessl B, editor. Berlin: Springer-Verlag; 1976.

28. Luhr HG. Compression plate osteosynthesis through the Luhr system. In: Krüger E, Schilli W, editors, Oral and maxillofacial traumatology, vol 1. Chicago: Quintessence; 1982.

29. Levy FE, Smith RW, Odland RM, et al. Monocortical miniplate fixation of mandibular fractures. Arch Otolaryngol Head Neck Surg 1991;117:149–54.

30. Choi BH, Kim KN, Kang HS, et al. Clinical and in vitro evaluation of mandibular angle fracture fixation with the two-miniplate system. Oral Surg 1995;79:692–5.

31. Choi BH, Yoo JH, Kim KN, et al. Stability testing of a two-miniplate fixation technique for mandibular angle fractures. An in vitro study. J Craniomaxillofac Surg 1995;23:123–5.

32. Fox AJ, Kellman RM. Mandibular angle fractures: two-miniplate fixation and complications. Arch Facial Plast Surg 2003;5:464–9.

33. Wald RM, Abemayor E, Zemplenyi J, et al. The transoral treatment of mandibular fractures using noncompression miniplates: a prospective study. Ann Plast Surg 1988;20:409–13.

34. Michelet FX, Deymes I, Dessus B, et al. Osteosynthesis with miniaturized plates in maxillofacial surgery. J Maxillofac Surg 1973;1:79–84.

35. Pape HD, Herzog M, Gerlach KL, et al. Der wandel der unterkeiferfrakturversorgung von 1950 bis 1980 am beispiel der Kglner Klinik. Dtsch Zahnarztl Z 1983;38:301–4 [German].

36. Pape HD, Gerlach KL. Le traitement des fractures des maxillaires chez l'enfant et l'adolescent. Rev Stomatol Chir Maxillofac 1980;81:280–4 [French].

37. Gerlach KL, Pape HD. Prinzip und indikation der miniplattenosteosynthbse. Dtsch Zahnaerztl Z 1980;35:346 [German].

38. Gerlach KL, Pape HD, Tuncer M, et al. Funktionsanalytische untersuchungen nach der miniplattenosteosynthese von unterkieferfrakturen. Dtsch Z Mund Kiefer Gesichts Chir 1982;6:57–61 [German].

39. Ewers R, Härle F. Biomechanics of the midface and mandibular fractures: Is a stable fixation necessary?. In: Hjorting-Hansen E, editor. Oral and maxillofacial surgery. Proceedings from the 8th International Conference on oral and maxillofacial surgery. Chicago: Quintessence; 1985. p. 207–11.

40. Ewers R, Härle F. Experimental and clinical results of new advances in the treatment of facial trauma. Plast Reconstr Surg 1985;75:25–31.

41. Feller K-U, Schneider M, Hlawitschka M, et al. Analysis of complications in fractures of the mandibular angle—a study with finite element computation and evaluation of data of 277 patients. J Craniomaxillofac Surg 2003;31:290–5.

42. Barry CP, Kearns GJ. Superior border plating technique in the management of isolated mandibular angle fractures: a retrospective study of 50 consecutive patients. J Oral Maxillofac Surg 2007;65: 1544–9.

43. Shetty V, McBrearty D, Fourney M, et al. Fracture line stability as a function of the internal fixation system: an in vitro comparison using a mandibular angle fracture model. J Oral Maxillofac Surg 1995;53: 791–801.

44. Alkan A, Celebi N, Ozden B, et al. Biomechanical comparison of different plating techniques in repair of mandibular angle fractures. Oral Surg Oral Med Oral Pathol Oral Radiol Endod 2007;104:752–6.

45. Wittenberg JM, Mukherjee DP, Smith BR, et al. Biomechanical evaluation of new fixation devices for mandibular angle fractures. Int J Oral Maxillofac Surg 1997;26:68–73.

46. Piffko J, Homann Ch, Schuon R, et al. Experimental study on the biomechanical stability of different internal fixators for use in the mandible. Mund Kiefer Gesichtschir 2003;7:1–6.

47. Feledy J, Caterson EJ, Steger S, et al. Treatment of mandibular angle fractures with a matrix miniplate: a preliminary report. Plast Reconstr Surg 2004;114: 1711–6.

48. Guimond C, Johnson JV, Marchena JM, et al. Fixation of mandibular angle fractures with a 2.0-mm

3-dimensional curved angle strut plate. J Oral Maxillofac Surg 2005;63:209–14.

49. Zix J, Lieger O, Iizuka T, et al. Use of straight and curved 3-dimensional titanium miniplates for fracture fixation at the mandibular angle. J Oral Maxillofac Surg 2007;65:1758–63.

50. Frost DE, Tucker MR, White RP. Small bone plate techniques for fixation of mandibular fractures. In: Tucker MR, Terry BC, White RP Jr, Sickels JE, editors. Rigid fixation for maxillofacial surgery. Philadelphia: JB Lippincott; 1991. p. 108–22.

51. Valentino J, Levy FE, Marentette LJ, et al. Intraoral monocortical miniplating of mandible fractures. Arch Otolaryngol Head Neck Surg 1994;120:605–12.

52. Schierle HP, Schmelzeisen R, Rahn B, et al. One- or two-plate fixation of mandibular angle fractures? J Craniomaxillofac Surg 1997;25:162–8.

53. Siddiqui A, Markose G, Moos KF, et al. One miniplate versus two in the management of mandibular angle fractures: a prospective randomised study. Br J Oral Maxillofac Surg 2007;45:223–5.

54. Cohen L. Further studies into the vascular architecture of the mandible. J Dent Res 1960;39:936–46.

55. Bradley JC. A radiological investigation into the age changes of the inferior dental artery. Br J Oral Surg 1975;14:82–90.

56. Hayter JP, Cawood JI. The functional case for miniplates in maxillofacial surgery. Int J Oral Maxillofac Surg 1993;22:91–6.

57. Gear AJ, Apasova E, Schmitz JP, et al. Treatment modalities for mandibular angle fractures. J Oral Maxillofac Surg 2005;63:655–63.

58. Theriot BA, Van Sickels JE, Triplett RB, et al. Intra-osseous wire fixation versus rigid osseous fixation of mandibular fractures: a preliminary report. J Oral Maxillofac Surg 1987;45:577–82.

59. Ellis E, Karas N. Treatment of mandibular angle fractures using two mini dynamic compression plates. J Oral Maxillofac Surg 1992;50:958–63.

60. Wagner WF, Neal DC, Alpert B, et al. Morbidity associated with extra oral open reduction of mandibular fractures. J Oral Surg 1979;37:97–100.

61. James RB, Fredrickson C, Kent JN, et al. Prospective study of mandibular fractures. J Oral Surg 1981;39:275–81.

62. Chuong R, Donoff RB, Guralnick WC, et al. A retrospective analysis of 327 mandibular fractures. J Oral Maxillofac Surg 1983;41:305–9.

63. Iizuka T, Lindqvist C, Hallikainen D, et al. Infection after rigid internal fixation of mandibular fractures. A clinical and radiological study. J Oral Maxillofac Surg 1991;49:585–93.

64. Anderson T, Alpert B. Experience with rigid fixation of mandibular fractures and immediate function. J Oral Maxillofac Surg 1992;50:555.

65. Schmelzeisen R, McIff T, Rahn B, et al. Further development of titanium miniplate fixation for mandibular fractures. Experience gained and questions raised from a prospective clinical pilot study with 2.0 mm fixation plates. J Craniomaxillofac Surg 1992;20:251–6.

66. Gabrielli MA, Gabrielli MF, Marcantonio E, et al. Fixation of mandibular fractures with 2.0-mm miniplates: review of 191 cases. J Oral Maxillofac Surg 2003;61:430–6.

67. Lamphier J, Ziccardi V, Ruvo A, et al. Complications of mandibular fractures in an urban teaching center. J Oral Maxillofac Surg 2003;61:745–9.

Management of Atrophic Mandible Fractures

Matthew J. Madsen, DMD[a],*, Richard H. Haug, DDS[b],
Bryan S. Christensen, DMD[c], Eron Aldridge, MD[b]

KEYWORDS

• Mandible • Fracture • Atrophic • Management • Elderly

The life expectancy of the elderly population has dramatically increased because of advances in health care and lifestyle changes.[1] Data from the US Census Bureau projects that by the year 2050 the population over the age of 65 will exceed 85 million people. Currently, 12.4% of the population is over 65 years old. That number is projected to increase to 20.7% by 2050.[2–4] If our ratios of patients were to parallel these figures, we could expect that by 2050 the percentage of our patients 65 years or older would be about double what it is today. Of course, patient ratios do not precisely follow ratios for the population as a whole. Even so, we can be certain that we will be seeing steadily increasing percentages of elderly patients as time goes on.

In the United States, longer life-expectancy has gone hand in hand with improved quality of life for many elderly people, compared to elderly Americans of the past. The older population enjoys more physical mobility and engages in more leisure activities than their counterparts of the past. As the elderly population continues to increase, oral and maxillofacial surgeons are faced with management of more difficult injuries in this group of patients. Among these injuries is the fracture of the atrophic edentulous mandible (**Fig. 1**). Many oral and maxillofacial surgeons are inexperienced in managing such injuries because they occur so rarely. In addition, because of this infrequency, surgical literature offers little updated information about management. This article reviews and evaluates the various past and current treatment methods and offers a look into possible improvements of some of these methods.

HISTORICAL PERSPECTIVE

Before the 1960s, management of the fractured atrophic mandible generally involved the use of closed treatment for reduction and stabilization or no treatment at all, otherwise known as "skillful neglect." The advent of internal fixation changed the way that such fractures are treated. Previous to use of rigid internal fixation, a number of other treatments were used to gain primary reduction and stability of these fractures. In some cases, the patient's denture was attached with circummandibular wires and used to stabilize the fracture (monomandibular fixation). If more stabilization was necessary, the upper denture could be fixed to the maxilla via direct wiring, circumzygomatic wiring, or pyriform aperture wiring and then the two dentures could be secured together using maxillomandibular fixation (MMF). However, MMF is poorly tolerated by many elderly individuals and can lead to other complications, such as decreased respiratory function as well as temporomandibular joint degeneration due to long periods of immobilization.[5] Nevertheless, this technique is still used by some surgeons when they feel that a conservative approach is necessary. The technique can be improved by using arch bars placed on the lower and upper dentures to provide MMF, or by uniting the

a Department of Oral and Maxillofacial Surgery, University of Louisville School of Dentistry, 501 S Preston Street, Louisville, Ste 334, Louisville, KY 40202, USA
b University of Kentucky College of Dentistry, Chandler Medical Center, 800 Rose Street, Lexington, KY 40536-0297, USA
c Oral and Maxillofacial Surgery, University of Oklahoma, Oklahoma City, OK, USA
* Corresponding author.
E-mail address: mjmads01@louisville.edu (M.J. Madsen).

Oral Maxillofacial Surg Clin N Am 21 (2009) 175–183
doi:10.1016/j.coms.2008.12.006

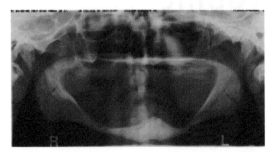

Fig. 1. A preoperative panoramic radiograph showing a bilateral atrophic edentulous mandibular "bucket handle" fracture.

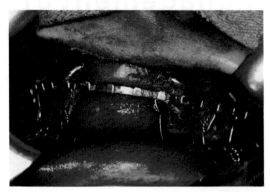

Fig. 3. Anterior opening for feeding created on the upper and lower members of a Gunning splint.

dentures into one unit with acrylic to decrease movement.[6,7]

Gunning splints historically have been used when complete dentures were not available. This technique is credited to Thomas Gunning, who used these splints to treat fractured jaws as early as 1863. Impressions are first made of the patient's maxilla and mandible. The mandibular cast is then cut and realigned when there is considerable displacement of the fracture. Separate units are made for both the maxillary and mandibular arches (**Fig. 2**). In an emergency situation, Gunning splints can be fabricated from disposable impression trays that are relined. An opening is always made in the anterior region for food to be ingested (**Fig. 3**). The use of Gunning splints is most favorable when extreme mandibular atrophy is not present and the fracture is not comminuted. Moreover, the fracture must lie in the denture-bearing area.

Gunning splints also have been used with open reduction techniques using nonrigid fixation, such as wires. Intraoperatively, the splints are first adapted to the edentulous ridges using warm gutta percha to line the interior surface. The upper splint is inserted first using 0.5 stainless steel wires passed through the alveolus (**Fig. 4**). The perialveolar wires can be supplemented with piriform or circumpalatal wires if the maxilla is atrophic. After the open reduction is done, the mandibular splint is secured by circumferential mandibular wires. At this time, the throat pack should be removed and the occlusion of the upper and lower splints verified. Stainless steel wires are then secured on hooks built into the splints and tightened to immobilize the upper and lower members in an MMF fashion (see **Fig. 3**).

The technique of circummandibular wiring has also been used without Gunning splints in cases of oblique fractures. This is accomplished by first doing an open approach to the fracture and then passing the circummandibular wires, which are twisted down to reduce the fractured segments (**Fig. 5**). However, this method may result in fracture instability as well as mucosal dehiscence over the wires.

However, the various closed techniques for treating fractures in the atrophic edentulous mandible using splints do not provide adequate resistance to the elevator muscles of mastication

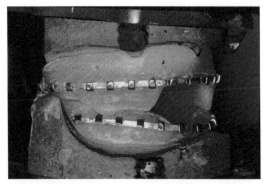

Fig. 2. Gunning splints with arch bars fabricated from acrylic on an articulator.

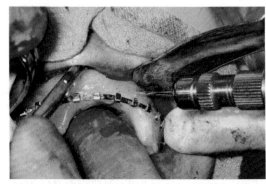

Fig. 4. A Gunning splint placed on the maxilla using peralveolar wiring.

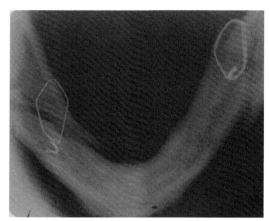

Fig. 5. Circummandibular wiring of oblique fractures.

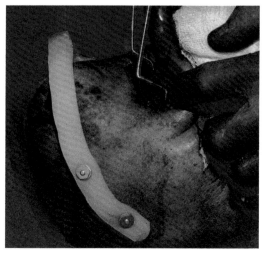

Fig. 6. Intraoperative placement of external fixator. Note the anterior and posterior pin connected by a transverse bar spanning the fracture.

and frequently lead to complications in healing. Therefore, they are generally not recommended.

Another closed method that may be used to treat edentulous mandibular fractures is external pin fixation. This technique is often indicated when the fracture is comminuted. One advantage to this method is that the placement of the pins does not require subperiosteal dissection. By maintaining the periosteal blood supply, healing is improved and further atrophy may be prevented. Two factors limit the use of this procedure. The first is the amount of bone available. It may be insufficient to accommodate the technique. The second is the appearance of the patient. Some patients are unwilling to accept such a disconcerting appearance during the course of treatment.

The concept of external pin fixation is simple in its application. When there is support from the contralateral side, an anterior and a posterior pin are placed with a transverse bar spanning the fracture (**Fig. 6**). Additional support is provided by at least one additional pin on either side of the fracture. Performing the procedure can be complicated when there is considerable edema present.

The underlying motivation for the development of new technology and improved surgical techniques is to address the abnormal anatomy often present in the fractured atrophic edentulous mandible. Blood supply from the surrounding periosteum plays an important role in healing, especially in the elderly and in injuries that include the mandibular canal. In some patients, the severe resorption may involve the mandibular canal, thus changing the blood supply pattern to the mandible. Sclerotic bone and poor circulation contribute to the high morbidity with atrophic mandibular fractures.[8,9]

Abnormal mandibular anatomy increases as the mandibular height decreases. Luhr and colleagues[10] classified atrophic edentulous mandibles as class 1 (16–20 mm), class 2 (11–15 mm), and class 3 ($\leq$10 mm). Cawood[11] further classified the resorption patterns of the alveolar bone following tooth extraction that occur in the anterior/posterior dimension. This resorption often results in a "knife edge" alveolar ridge, which is then followed by vertical resorption until the basal bone of the mandible is encountered. Once minimal alveolar bone is present, the fracture becomes more difficult to treat using closed techniques.

CURRENT THERAPY

There is still controversy concerning the most appropriate treatment of a fracture of the edentulous atrophic mandible. There are proponents of a conservative approach, such as a closed reduction technique, and there are advocates for a more invasive open reduction procedure (**Tables 1** and **2**). Those of the conservative philosophy have several reasons why they believe a less invasive model should be followed. As the patient loses dentition, there is a successive loss of osseous structure and a decreased blood supply to the area.[11] The reduction of vascularity can then lead to a diminished ability of the fracture to heal properly and contribute to a possible malunion or nonunion.[6,12] Bruce and Ellis[13] reported that a decrease in the height of the mandible increases the likelihood of complications related to fracture healing.

Furthermore, in the conservative view, a closed reduction technique is much less likely to result in complications than the use of the

Table 1
Closed reduction techniques for atrophic edentulous mandible fractures

Technique	Description	Advantages	Disadvantages
Preexisting mandibular denture with circummandibular wiring	Patient's denture used to stabilize mandibular fracture	If a maxillary denture exists, arch bars can be used for maxillomandibular fixation, while circumzygomatic and piriform wires will stabilize the maxillary denture	Nonrigid fixation; compliance issues; maxillomandibular fixation in the elderly, poorly tolerated in infirm patient
Gunning splint	Acrylic maxillary and mandibular prosthesis with an oral opening and circummandibular wiring	Oral opening allows for food intake; single unit device	Fracture mobility a concern if circummandibular wiring placed too close to fracture site; nonrigid fixation; compliance issues
External pin fixation appliances	A variety of devices that place fixation pins into the mandible for stabilization of fractures	May be placed at the bedside; no maxillomandibular fixation needed; no compliance issues; useful when patient cannot tolerate an extensive open operation	Requires good quantity of mandibular bone for placement of fixation pins; nonrigid fixation; potential damage to inferior alveolar nerve; unwillingness of some patients to accept disconcerting appearance
"No treatment"/ soft diet	Soft diet, close observation, no surgical intervention	May be appropriate in minimally displaced, unilateral fractures, or in patients with severe systemic illness or injury	Potential for a dysfunctional endpoint

open technique on an elderly patient. This is because of the decrease of contacting bone surface area in the mandible. With less bone surface area to work with, more technical precision is required in an open reduction, especially if plates and screws are used. Unless the surgeon is prepared to meet such high precision demands, a closed reduction technique is more prudent.

Another problem with the open technique, according to the conservative opinion, stems from the likelihood that older patients tend to have a variety of systemic diseases and significant health problems. These health issues increase the chance of morbidity and mortality in these patients. A longer, more complicated open reduction procedure may increase such risks. Undergoing general anesthesia alone is a risk factor in the geriatric patient, with morbidity occurring four times more often in an older patient than in a younger patient.[6,14]

Open reduction involves direct exposure of the fracture site and placement of internal fixation to prevent movement and allow healing by primary intention. Due to the absence of teeth, malocclusion is not a consideration and the primary consideration becomes adequate reduction of the bony segments. Open reduction of an atrophic edentulous mandible body fracture can be accomplished via a transoral or an extraoral approach. The submandibular approach can be used to access a body fracture in most instances. Anatomic concerns about the facial artery and marginal mandibular branch of the facial nerve must be addressed in the dissection when using such an approach. The transoral approach can be employed to gain access to most edentulous mandibular fractures. The body and symphysis regions of the mandible have good access and visibility. However, the ramus, inferior border, and angle present problems because access can be limited. The two biggest risk factors with the transoral route are lip malposition and mental nerve damage. The greatest advantage of the transoral approach is that it does not leave a visible scar. Toma and colleagues[15] found that a comparison of transoral versus extraoral approaches in dentate mandible fractures resulted in different complication rates. Clinical experience with patients subgrouped into transoral versus extraoral approaches suggests that the transoral approach has a greater association with infection and nonunion. It seems reasonable that these complications in dentate patients would be similar in the atrophic edentulous mandible patients.

Once the fracture is accessed and reduced, regardless of the approach, there are three common methods of fixation: a 2.4-mm reconstruction plate, titanium mesh, or a locking miniplate. The 2.4-mm reconstruction plate is strong enough to overcome the functional load as well as to counteract the masticatory forces. However, the screws in these large plates may cause another fracture upon placement. Also, because the bone is weak and fragile, the screws can fail by stripping the bone, which leads to inflammation and bony necrosis. Large bicortical screws can cause injury to the inferior alveolar nerve leading to a lower lip dysesthesia.[16,17] In spite of these disadvantages, a reconstruction plate, because of its ability to provide primary stability, is the AO/ASIF (Arbeitsgemeinschaft für Osteosynthesefragen/Association for the Study of Internal Fixation) method of treating an atrophic edentulous mandible fracture. Also, a reconstruction plate satisfies the goal of the patient to return to immediate function, while resisting hardware fracture.[16]

A titanium mesh crib with a simultaneous iliac crest, anterior tibial, rib, or calvarial bone graft is another approach to augmenting the edentulous ridge and stabilizing the fracture. The advantages include the use of an autogenous graft to enhance bone density at the surgical site. However, such a graft creates the possibility of morbidity at the donor site, such as the hip or the lower leg, with gait disturbances. Graft infection, resorption, and nonunion are additional drawbacks to this procedure.

A few surgeons advocate the use of miniplates. The theory behind the use of this type of plate is "the smaller the better," the idea being that a small plate is sufficient for the purpose and, because it is small, is less likely to result in periosteal stripping than a larger plate.[18] An advantage of this approach is the ease of placement. Advocates of this technique also argue that it is beneficial because miniplates do not need as much bone density as a reconstruction plate to achieve rigid internal fixation. However, Eyrich[17] noted that miniplates are subject to failure due to inability of the plates to withstand the load placed on them by the maxillomandibular forces.

Because of the decreased surface area of bone, we do not advocate the use of a lag screw to fix and compress the bone fragments on either side of the fracture in an atrophic edentulous mandible. This technique is primarily reserved for the oblique, horizontally directed angle fracture or for parasymphyseal fractures in mandibles that have adequate height.

FUTURE DEVELOPMENTS

One of the most rapidly developing areas of research involves surgical fracture repair using novel materials or improved plating techniques. One technique suggested is to place a 2.4-mm reconstruction plate on the inferior border of the atrophic mandible using an extraoral approach (**Fig. 7**).[19] This avoids complications associated with placement of a plate on the lateral border of the atrophic mandible. A modified apron incision is used to expose the inferior border of the mandible, which provides good visualization for plate adaptation. The plate is then secured by locking screws in the standard fashion (**Figs. 8 and 9**). The advantages of this technique are threefold. First, by using an extraoral approach, the likelihood of wound dehiscence and infection decreases, and lack of soft tissue coverage is less likely to be problem.[15] Second, the biomechanics of a reconstruction plate placed on the inferior border of the mandible is similar to that of a reconstruction plate placed on the lateral border.[19] Both approaches using reconstruction plates (inferior border or lateral border) have been shown to exceed the demands of functional loading placed on the edentulous atrophic mandible and plating system when simulated in vitro. Third, the patient may continue to wear a prosthesis, which can further stabilize the fracture.

Another technique that has been described to reconstruct the atrophic mandible fracture involves the use of a resorbable mesh rather than a titanium mesh as a containment system to rebuild the ridge in the site of atrophy using autogenous bone grafts.[20] The mesh is contoured to encompass the defect and then is secured by 1.5-mm tacks. This material offers several advantages: (1) It maintains the shape and location of the graft during the consolidation phase; (2) it does not require a second surgery to remove the material; and (3) it can be shaped into different configurations to follow the contour of the mandible.[20] This procedure also involves stabilization of the fracture with a reconstruction plate.

Table 2
Open reduction and internal fixation techniques for atrophic edentulous mandible fractures

Technique	Description	Advantages	Disadvantages
Pencil bone plate	2.0-mm titanium osteosynthesis miniplate with a reinforced midregion designed for the atrophic mandible	18 of 20 edentulous patients with mandibular heights ranging from "10 mm or less" to 20 mm showed fibrous healing without complication;[25] allows unrestricted wearing of dentures, theoretically improving nutritional status	New design without lengthy track record of performance
Open reduction and internal fixation with miniplate	After exposure and reduction of bony fragments, generally a 3-hole-per-segment, 2.0-mm titanium miniplate is fixed to fracture site using 6.0-mm monocortical titanium screws (variation is common)	Small size of miniplate; efficient and easy to use	In the atrophic edentulous mandible, miniplates show significantly less resistance to displacement when used for fractures in mandibles under 30 mm in height
Open reduction and internal fixation with titanium mesh and bone graft	After exposure and reduction of bony fragments, titanium mesh is cut to size, adapted, and fixed in place with monocortical screws, overlapping the fracture by 20 mm on each side	Rate of bony union without complications is 70%;[26] autologous bone grafts similarly held securely with the mesh	Patients may have increased risk for infection and intraoral wound dehiscence; rate of minor complication (hematoma) is 20%[25]
Open reduction and internal fixation with Mennen plate	A supraperiosteal, paraskeletal stainless steel bone-clamping device placed after open reduction of mandibular fracture	An alternative to conventional screw-retained plates for fixation of atrophic mandible fractures where screws may cause sensory disturbance or worsen jaw fracture	Bulky appliance
Autogenous primary rib graft	Rib harvested for use as a splint in repair of atrophic edentulous mandible fractures	Enlargement of the bony ridge; one study showed all 15 rib-grafted patients achieved bony union and were subsequently able to wear dentures;[27] reduces the risk of pseudoarthrosis and facilitates subsequent prosthetic rehabilitation	Rib harvesting may increase the risk of pulmonary atelectasis and pneumonia, but can be minimized using local anesthetic infusion at harvest site

(continued on next page)

Table 2
(continued)

Technique	Description	Advantages	Disadvantages
Compression osteosynthesis	The Vitallium minicompression system may be used in the atrophic edentulous mandible with self-tapping, bicortically anchored screws	One study has shown that in 96.5% of fractures, an uncomplicated, solid, bony union was achieved;[10] no maxillomandibular fixation necessary	Horizontal plating is discouraged; sensory disturbances always a potential problem in bone plating of mandibular fractures, but may be more common in the atrophic mandible, although inferior placement should avoid this problem
Reconstruction plate	After exposure and reduction of bony fragments, generally a 2.4-mm titanium reconstruction plate is fixed in place with 3 bicortical titanium screws per segment (variation is common)	At high loads, atrophic mandibles (10 mm in height) repaired with reconstruction plates provide resistance to displacement equivalent to that found in mandibles 40 mm in height repaired with miniplates;[28] may be less susceptible to fatigue and may show a reduced tendency for screws to loosen under cyclic loading, which decreases the rate of postoperative infection and failure	Long bicortical screws may violate the inferior alveolar nerve; large bicortical screws may create a jaw fracture; large plating systems require wider stripping of the periosteum; less periosteal contact with bone after plate placement

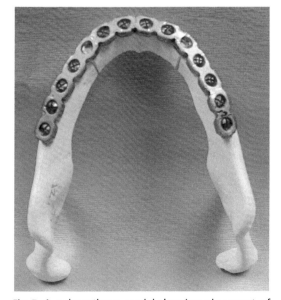

Fig. 7. A polyurethane model showing placement of a 2.4-mm reconstruction plate on the inferior border of the mandible.

The use of alloplastic materials instead of autogenous grafts to reconstruct the atrophic mandible is increasingly favored because it avoids the use of autogenous graft sites and thus possible morbidity

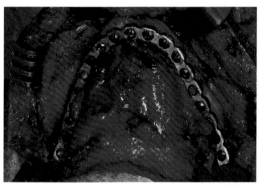

Fig. 8. An intraoperative photograph of the surgical approach and contour of the reconstruction plate to the inferior border of the mandible.

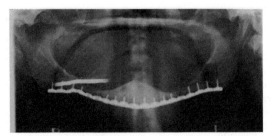

Fig. 9. A postoperative panoramic radiograph showing plate adaptation to the mandible and reduction of the fractures bilaterally.

associated with a second surgical site for autogenous bone grafting. These alloplastic materials include hydroxyapatite, tricalcium phosphate, glass ceramics, and glass carbonate.[21] These materials and their emerging uses each have limitations. These materials vary depending on the nature of the scaffold (ie, permanent or biodegradable; naturally occurring or synthetic), biocompatibility characteristics, osteoconductivity characteristics, ability to integrate, porosity, and mechanical compatibility.[22] Injectable calcium phosphate cements have been shown to be biocompatible and have applications to the atrophic mandible.[21] Calcium phosphates have high plasticity initially and then harden in situ to develop great compressive strengths. Because of these properties, calcium phosphates can be used for ridge augmentation procedures. The overall goal in placing these materials is to guide the physiologic and biologic response during repair of the fracture. The application of these materials is appealing when considering health complications that prolong healing and can lead to nonunion and other associated complications.

Recent attempts to develop a tissue-engineered scaffold with both osteoconductivity and osteoinductivity have included loading osteoinductive proteins, or osteogenic cells, or a combination of both onto the traditional bioactive materials. Covalent linking of compounds, such as bone morphogenic protein 2, to resorbable plates has shown promise in promoting fracture repair. Covalent linking of compounds to plates represents a novel method for delivering concentrated levels of growth factors to a specific site and potentially extending their half-lives.[23] Future advances in bone regeneration will likely incorporate therapies that use the tools of gene therapy and tissue engineering to mimic aspects of these natural biological processes.[24]

SUMMARY

Many surgeons find the repair of the fractured atrophic edentulous mandible to be difficult. As the population ages, we can anticipate treating more of these fractures, which means surgeons need a good understanding of the advantages and drawbacks of each potential treatment so that the most appropriate treatment is used to achieve the best functional result. History has demonstrated that a number of treatments are practical. However, it has also shown us that there is room to improve the treatment approaches for this specific fracture type. As plating systems and bone regeneration therapies improve, the outcome following treatment of the fractured atrophic mandible will also likely improve.

REFERENCES

1. Marciani RD. Critical systemic and psychosocial considerations in management of trauma in the elderly. Oral Surg Med Oral Pathol Oral Radiol Endod 1999;87:272–80.
2. Available at: http://www.census.gov/ipc/www/usinterimproj. Accessed July 11, 2008.
3. Perren SM, Allgöwer M. Manual of internal fixation: techniques recommended by the AO-ASIF Group. 3rd edition. Germany: Springer Verlag; 1991. p. 16.
4. Kushner GM, Alpert B. Management of mandibular body fractures. Atlas Oral Maxillofac Surg Clin North Am 1997;5(1):63–4.
5. Zide MF, Ducic Y. Fibula microvascular free tissue reconstruction of the severely comminuted atrophic mandible fracture case report. J Cranio-Maxillofac Surg 2003;31:296–8.
6. Scott RF. Oral and maxillofacial trauma in the geriatric patient. In: Fonseca RJ, Walker RV, editors. Oral and maxillofacial trauma, 2nd edition, vol. 2. Philadelphia: Saunders; 1997. p. 1045–72.
7. Spina AM, Marciani RD. Mandibular fractures. In: Fonseca RJ, Marciani RD, editors. Oral and maxillofacial surgery, vol. 3. Philadelphia: Saunders; 2000. p. 103–7.
8. Ellis E. Treatment methods for fractures of the mandibular angle. J Craniomaxillofac Trauma 1999;28:243–52.
9. McGregor AD, MacDonald DG. Age changes in the human inferior alveolar artery—a histological study. Br J Oral Maxillofac Surg 1989;27:371–4.
10. Luhr HG, Reidick T, Merten HA. Results of treatment of fractures of the atrophic edentulous mandible by compression plating: a retrospective evaluation of 84 consecutive cases. J Oral Maxillofac Surg 1996;54:250–5.
11. Cawood JI, Howell RA. A classification of the edentulous jaws. Int J Oral Maxillofac Surg 1988;17:232–6.
12. Buchbinder D. Treatment of fractures of the edentulous mandible, 1943 to 1993: a review of the literature. J Oral Maxillofac Surg 1993;51:1174–80.

13. Bruce RA, Ellis E. The second Chalmers J. Lyons Academy study of fractures of the edentulous mandible. J Oral Maxillofac Surg 1993;51:904–11.

14. Jones RL. Anesthesia risk in the geriatric patient. In: McLeskey CH, editor. Perioperative geriatrics: problems in anesthesia, vol. 3. Philadelphia: Lippincott; 1989. p. 529.

15. Toma VS, Mathog RH, Toma RS, et al. Transoral versus extraoral reduction of mandible fractures: a comparison of complication rates and other factors. Otolaryngol Head Neck Surg 2003;128:215–9.

16. Marciani RD. Invasive management of the fractured atrophic edentulous mandible. J Oral Maxillofac Surg 2001;59:792–5.

17. Eyrich GK, Gratz KW. Surgical treatment of fractures of the edentulous mandible. J Oral Maxillofac Surg 1997;55:1081–7.

18. Thaller SR. Fractures of the edentulous mandible: a retrospective review. J Craniofac Surg 1993;4:91–4.

19. Madsen MJ, Haug RH. A biomechanical comparison of two techniques for reconstructing atrophic edentulous mandible fractures. J Oral Maxillofac Surg 2006;64:457–65.

20. Louis P, Holmes J, Fernandes R. Resorbable mesh as a containment system in reconstruction of the atrophic mandible fracture. J Oral Maxillofac Surg 2004;62:719–23.

21. Wolff KD, Swaid S, Nolte D, et al. Degradable injectable bone cement in maxillofacial surgery: indications and clinical experience in 27 patients. J Craniomaxillofac Surg 2004;32:71–9.

22. El-Ghannam A. Bone reconstruction: from bioceramics to tissue engineering. Expert Rev Med Devices 2005;2:87–101.

23. Shibuya TY, Wadhwa A, Nguyen KH, et al. Linking of bone morphogenetic protein-2 to resorbable fracture plates for enhancing bone healing. Laryngoscope 2005;115:2232–7.

24. Franceschi RT. Biological approaches to bone regeneration by gene therapy. J Dent Res 2005;84:1093–103.

25. Seper L, Piffko J, Joos U, et al. Treatment of fractures of the atrophic mandible in the elderly. J Am Geriatr Soc 2004;52(9):1583–4.

26. Shug T, Rodemer H, Neupert W, et al. Treatment of complex mandibular fractures using titanium mesh. J Craniomaxillofac Surg 2000;28:235–7.

27. Newman I. The role of autogenous primary rib grafts in treating fractures of the atrophic edentulous mandible. Br J Oral Maxillofac Surg 1995;33:381–7.

28. Sikes JW, Smith BR, Mukherjee DP. An in vitro study of the effect of bony buttressing on fixation strength of a fractured atrophic edentulous mandible model. J Oral Maxillofac Surg 2000;58:56–62.

Management of Comminuted Fractures of the Mandible

Brian Alpert, DDS*, Paul S. Tiwana, DDS, MD, MS,
George M. Kushner, DMD, MD

KEYWORDS

• Fractures • Comminuted • Mandible

Comminuted mandible fractures are complex injuries that are generally the result of a significant impact on a localized area of the jaw by either a high-speed collision or a high-speed projectile. Most series of mandibular fractures report 5% to 7% as being comminuted. In a comminuted fracture, the bone is shattered. Most of these fractures are exposed to the mouth or skin. Gunshots are common causes. These complex injuries are difficult to treat and have a high complication rate.

TRADITIONAL MANAGEMENT

The management of comminuted mandibular fractures has evolved. Traditionally, one never opened the comminuted fracture so as to avoid devitalizing the bone fragments, which would ultimately sequester. With few exceptions, these cases were managed with closed techniques based on maxillomandibular fixation (MMF), splints, or both.[1–8] Proximal segment control, when necessary, was accomplished with skeletal pin fixation (**Figs. 1** and **2**). Obviously, if the fracture was secondary to a gunshot injury, there were also blast injury and cavitation considerations in management, depending on the type of firearm and projectiles involved. Most civilian gunshot wounds are secondary to fairly low velocity handguns or shotguns and do not have the cavitation and shock effects of the modern high- and ultra-high–velocity military projectiles. As such, civilian gunshot wounds are usually amenable to more aggressive management.[8]

Traditional management of a gunshot wound of the mandible, following management of any

airway or bleeding problems, would be to rule out vascular injury. Once done with neck exploration, and later with carotid angiograms, it is now accomplished with a CT angiogram. Debridement of both hard and soft tissue was based on the type of gunshot wound, but generally involved removal of bone fragments devoid of soft tissue attachment (and thus blood supply), with care being taken not to strip the periosteum from vital fragments. The rule of thumb was to remove only that bone that was flushed out with aggressive irrigation. Any bone still with soft tissue attachment was considered potentially viable. Shattered teeth as well as nonrestorable teeth associated with the fracture were also removed and soft tissue closure of the wound would be attempted. The principles of debridement and closure of these injuries are well established.[9,10] Application of MMF and an external fixater for proximal segment control, or an external fixator alone if the patient was edentulous, provided reduction and fixation of the bone fragments (**Figs. 3** and **4**). Further debridement was often necessary when drainage developed and additional fragments sloughed (see **Fig. 3**). Finally, after drainage ceased and the wound was closed, signifying initial consolidation of the comminuted fragments, reconstruction of any remaining defects was done in one or more stages.[11,12] Rehabilitation of function followed.

Obviously, this type of management was rather prolonged, with a treatment time of months (and sometimes years) rather than weeks. Yet, it was considered the gold standard for 70 years. It is well documented and illustrated by the US Navy

University of Louisville School of Dentistry, KY 40292, USA
* Corresponding author.
E-mail address: brian.alpert@louisville.edu (B. Alpert).

Oral Maxillofacial Surg Clin N Am 21 (2009) 185–192
doi:10.1016/j.coms.2008.12.002

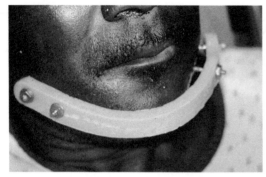

Fig. 1. Joe Hall Morris appliance for comminuted fracture of the symphysis.

Vietnam War experience.[12] The introduction of rigid fixation techniques which have dramatically shortened the course of treatment, raise the question of which form of treatment is preferable.

CONTEMPORARY MANAGEMENT

Rigid internal fixation with function during convalescence came into general use in Europe in the 1970s.[13–17] As part of this regimen, new techniques evolved for the treatment of comminuted fractures

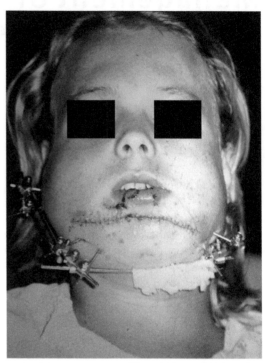

Fig. 2. Roger Anderson appliance controlling multiple comminuted mandibular fractures.

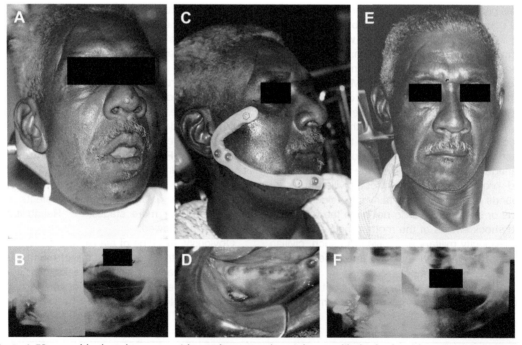

Fig. 3. A 58-year-old edentulous man with gunshot wound to right mandibular body with extensive contamination and comminution managed with external fixation. (*A*) Initial presentation. (*B*) Panoramic radiograph showing the comminuted fracture. (*C*) External fixator adapted to provide maxillomandibular fixation via attachment to the zygoma. (*D*) Sloughing bone fragments. (*E*) Final appearance at 2 months. (*F*) Panoramic radiograph showing final result.

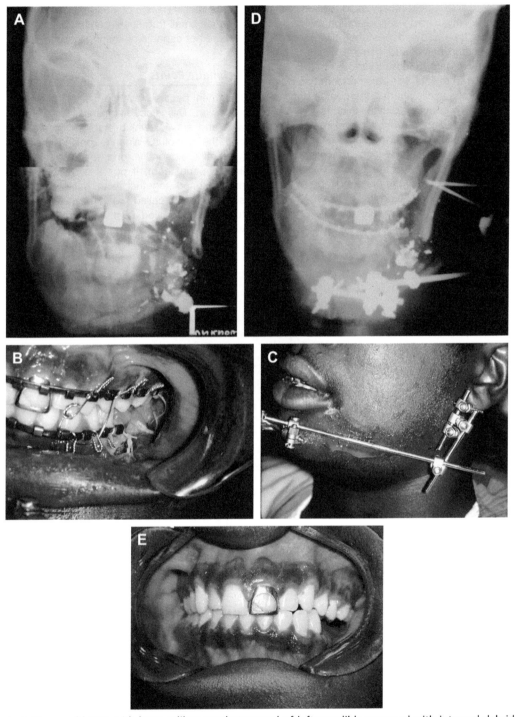

Fig. 4. A 21-year-old man with large-caliber gunshot wound of left mandible managed with intraoral debridement, MMF, and external fixation with a Roger Anderson device. (*A*) Radiograph demonstrating extensive comminution. (*B*) MMF following conservative intraoral debridement of bone and tooth fragments. (*C*) Control of proximal fragment with Roger Anderson appliance. (*D*) Radiograph showing external fixator. (*E*) Final occlusion.

of the mandible. Conceptually, rigid fixation of the fragments minimized sequestration while at the same time allowed postoperative function. The technique came into general use in North America by the late 1980s and various investigators have reported results[18–27] This concept has done much to dramatically shorten the course of treatment for these complex, difficult injuries (**Fig. 5**).

Essentially, an open reduction and internal fixation of the entire comminuted fracture complex is performed using load-bearing osteosynthesis. Any defects are bone grafted, as necessary. In this particular protocol, the plate must be big and strong enough to withstand the functional forces on this area of the mandible. Stabilization by compression or any other form of load-sharing osteosynthesis is obviously contraindicated because small fragments cannot be compressed and are not capable of sharing loads.

Technique Points

Treatment begins with rigid fixation of the teeth in occlusion. This is accomplished with arch bars or wire and acrylic, which stabilize both the teeth and the alveolus. When exposing the fracture (generally extraorally), one needs to maintain the lingual periosteum, if possible. Small fragments are fastened together with miniplates and lag screws, the so-called "simplification" of the fracture. The simplified segments are then bridged with a locking reconstruction plate and three or

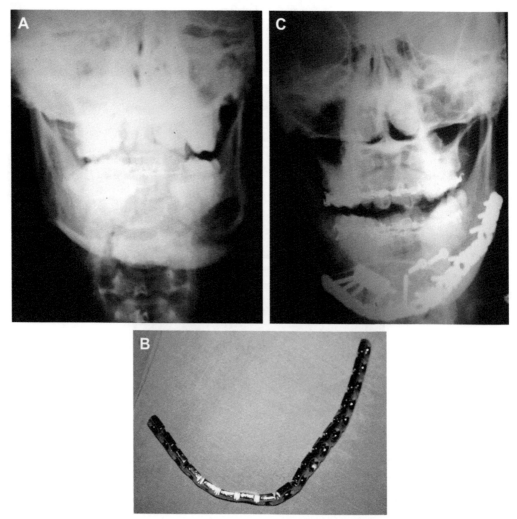

Fig. 5. (*A*) Early example of management of a comminuted mandibular fracture with a stainless steel reconstruction plate and lag screws, allowing postoperative function. Radiograph showing comminuted fracture of mandible. (*B*) Stainless steel 2.7-mm reconstruction plate. (*C*) Radiograph showing results of open reduction and rigid fixation. Note the absence of MMF allowing postoperative function.

four screws on either side of the fracture ends (**Fig. 6**). Most experience has been gained with 2.7-mm reconstruction or 2.4-mm locking plates, but the heavier variety of 2.0-mm locking plate is now becoming popular. It remains to be seen if the latter will offer sufficient strength and stability. MMF is released after plating, allowing at least limited function.

Defect Fractures

Some comminuted fractures result in defects because detached bone fragments were removed.

With rigid fixation, there is no micromovement to stimulate callus formation. Therefore, these defects will not fill in with new bone and thus need to be grafted.[15] If the overlying soft tissue is healthy, and wound closure is possible, grafting can take place at the time of initial repair (**Fig. 7**). The preferred graft material is autogenous particulate bone and marrow because of its rapid revascularization and resistance to infection. The preferred donor site is the tibia. If there are other considerations, such as inadequate wound coverage or potential cavitation necrosis, as

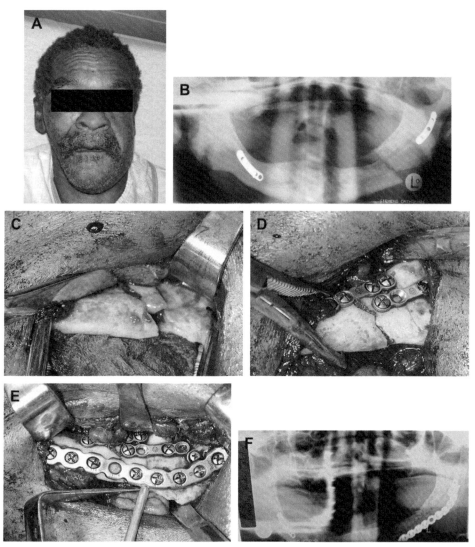

Fig. 6. A 62-year-old man who sustained a comminuted fracture of the left posterior body of the mandible from a beating with a pipe. (*A*) Initial presentation. (*B*) Panoramic radiograph showing plate from treatment of a previous treatment and new fracture of left body. (*C*) Extensive comminution seen when fracture is exposed. (*D*) Reduction of fractures and "simplification" with miniplates. (*E*) Application of locking reconstruction plate. Note at least three screws on either side of the fracture. (*F*) Postoperative radiograph.

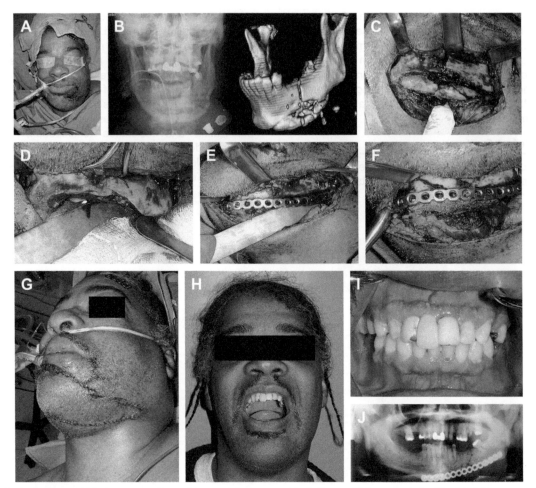

Fig. 7. A 22-year-old man presenting with a gunshot wound to left mandible managed with debridement and primary reconstruction with locking reconstruction plate and a particulate bone and marrow graft. (*A*) Presentation in the operating room. (*B*) Posteroanterior radiograph and three-dimensional CT scan of comminuted fracture of the mandible. (*C*) Exposure of fractures following placement of MMF. (*D*) Debridement of inferior border. (*E*) Application of locking reconstruction plate. (*F*) Reconstruction with tibial bone graft. (*G*) View of wound closure. (*H*) Mouth opening at 2 weeks. (*I*) Final occlusion. (*J*) Postoperative panoramic radiograph.

occurs in some gunshot wounds, the defect can be grafted later.

DISCUSSION

Comminuted fractures of the mandible have long been managed successfully with closed techniques relying on MMF and external devices. The military experience of World War I, World War II, the Korean War, and the Vietnam War not only established, but reinforced and perfected the principles and techniques of closed management.[11,12] Yet, even with ultimate successful outcomes, these closed techniques result in long (months to years) treatment times, with attendant disability.

Properly executed rigid fixation has proven to be a great advance in the management of comminuted fractures of the mandible. The outcomes are improved and the course of treatment is significantly shortened. Elimination of postoperative MMF allows function and does much to minimize the restriction from scarring, which often occurs with conservative closed treatment. Indeed, the patient usually remains functional, even during complications.

However, there is still a place for conservative treatment. When postoperative function or shortening the course of treatment are not an issue, as in a patient with a significant head injury, conservative treatment with closed techniques offers a realistic alternative to a major surgical procedure (**Fig. 8**). Likewise, if the surgical team is not well versed in the nuances of rigid internal fixation, or the necessary equipment is not

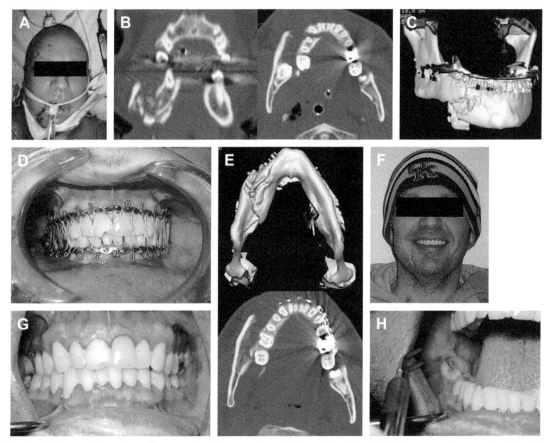

Fig. 8. A 38-year-old police officer involved in an automobile accident in which his car went over a bridge. He sustained severe head injuries and was in the intensive care unit in a vegetative state. Although he had a severely displaced, comminuted fracture of the mandible, only a closed reduction with MMF was permitted 1 month following the injury. He ultimately woke up and was rehabilitated. (*A*) Presentation 1 month after the accident. Note intracranial pressure monitor. (*B*) CT scans showing the displaced, comminuted fractures of the mandible. (*C*) Three-dimensional CT scan showing the fractures. (*D*) Treatment with arch bars and elastics. (*E*) Postreduction regular CT scan and three-dimensional CT scan showing that there is still displacement. (*F*) Appearance of patient 9 months after closed reduction. (*G*) Occlusion at 9 months. (*H*) Mouth opening at 9 months.

available, it is far better to do simple closed treatment. It has stood the test of time and achieves more than adequate results in most cases.

REFERENCES

1. Kazanjian VH, Converse JM. Surgical treatment of facial injuries. Baltimore (MD): Williams & Wilkins Co.; 1959. p. 179.
2. Rowe NL, Killey HC. Fractures of the facial skeleton. Baltimore (MD): Williams & Wilkins Co.; 1968. p. 23.
3. Alpert B, Martinez S. Skeletal trauma of the face. In: Richardson JD, Polk HC Jr, Flint LM, editors. Trauma: clinical care and pathophysiology. Chicago: Year Book Medical Publishers, Inc.; 1987. p. 278.
4. Bruce R, Fonseca RJ. Mandibular fractures. In: Fonseca RJ, Walker RV, editors, Oral and maxillofacial trauma, vol 1. Philadelphia: WB Saunders Co.; 1991. p. 391.
5. Mainous EG, Sazima HF, Stump ET, et al. Early care. In: Kelly JF, editor. Management of war injuries to the jaws and related structures. Washington (DC): US Government Printing Office; 1977. p. 74–8, Chap IV.
6. Walker RV, Frame JW. Civilian maxillo-facial gunshot injuries. Int J Oral Surg 1984;13:263.
7. Neupert EA, Boyd SB. Retrospective analysis of low-velocity gunshot wounds to the mandible. Oral Surg 1991;72:383.
8. Osborne TE, Bays RA. Pathophysiology and management of gunshot wounds to the face. In: Fonseca RH, Walker RV, editors, Oral and maxillofacial trauma, vol 1. Philadelphia: WB Saunders Co; 1991. p. 687.
9. Osbon DB. Early treatment of soft tissue injuries of the face. J Oral Surg 1969;27:480–7.

10. Joy ED. Early care of maxillofacial missile wounds. J Oral Surg 1973;31:475–8.
11. Osbon DB. Intermediate and reconstructive care of maxillofacial missile wounds. J Oral Surg 1973;31:429–37.
12. Kelly JF. Management of war injuries to the jaw and related structures. Washington, DC: US Government Printing Office; 1977.
13. Schilli W. Compression osteosynthesis. J Oral Surg 1977;35:802.
14. Champy M, Lodde JP, Schmitt R, et al. Mandibular osteosynthesis by miniature screwed plates via a buccal approach. J Maxillofac Surg 1978;6:21.
15. Spiessl B. Stable internal fixation. In: Mathog RH, editor. Maxillofacial trauma. Baltimore (MD): Williams and Wilkins Co; 1984. p. 162–76, CH 11B.
16. Spiessl B. New concepts in maxillofacial bone surgery. Berlin: Springer-Verlag; 1976.
17. Spiessl B. Comminuted fractures. In: Internal fixation of the mandible. Berlin: Springer-Verlag; 1989. p. 235–40.
18. Klotch D. Use of rigid internal fixation in the repair of complex and comminuted mandible fractures. Otolaryngol Clin North Am 1987;20:495.
19. Prein J, Kellman RM. Rigid internal fixation of mandibular fractures: basics of AO techniques. Otolaryngol Clin North Am 1987;20:441.
20. Assael LA. Results in rigid internal fixation in highly comminuted fractures of the mandible. J Oral Maxillofac Surg 1989;47:119.
21. Buchbinder D. Use of rigid internal fixation in the treatment of mandibular fractures. Oral Maxillofac Surg Clin North Am 1990;2(1):41–54.
22. Anderson T, Alpert B. Experience with rigid fixation of mandibular fractures and immediate function. J Oral Maxillofac Surg 1992;50:555.
23. Smith BR, Johnson JV. Rigid fixation of comminuted mandibular fractures. J Oral Maxillofac Surg 1993; 51:1320.
24. Assael LA. Treatment of comminuted fractures of the mandible. Atlas Oral Maxillofac Surg Clin North Am Mar 1977;5(1).
25. Ellis E III, Muniz O, Anand K. Treatment considerations for comminuted mandibular fractures. J Oral Maxillofac Surg 2003;61:861–70.
26. Finn RA. Treatment of comminuted mandibular fractures by closed reduction. J Oral Maxillofac Surg 1996;54:320–7.
27. Smith BR, Teenier TJ. Treatment of comminuted mandibular fractures by open reduction and rigid internal fixation. J Oral Maxillofac Surg 1996;54: 328–31.

Management of Condylar Process Fractures

Daniel M. Laskin, DDS, MS

KEYWORDS

- Fractures • Condylar process • Child • Adult
- Open reduction • Closed reduction

Clinicians generally agree about the treatment of fractures in most regions of the mandible. However, considerable controversy continues regarding the management of fractures of the condylar process because the occlusion cannot be used to reestablish the alignment of the segments, which can only be accomplished through an open reduction. Meanwhile, concerns remain about the potential risk of injury to the facial nerve when operating in this region, despite the various approaches to the area that have been developed. Therefore, the crucial question is whether precise alignment of the segments is necessary to provide the best functional results. In attempting to answer this question, one needs to be reminded that some condylar process fractures clearly call for open treatment and others clearly call for closed treatment. For example, sometimes displacement is minimal, and sometimes there are intracapsular fractures in which the condylar fragment is too small to be plated. For such cases, everyone would agree that closed treatment is indicated. Conversely, when there is a need to establish a solid mandible as a base for correcting associated midface fractures, or when there is interference with establishing a proper occlusion, everyone would agree that open reduction might be necessary. These are cases in which the choice of open or closed treatment is clear. However, in many situations the choice is not so obvious and the clinician must carefully weigh the benefits and risks of each approach.

In reviewing the literature, one finds conflicting evidence as to whether the open reduction of condylar process fractures leads to better condylar movement, better occlusion, and less facial asymmetry. For example, in a study on mandibular movement following open or closed treatment of condylar process fractures, Steish-Scholz and colleagues[1] found that, although the mean condylar paths were consistently shorter in patients treated by closed reduction, the differences were significant only for movements without tooth contact and that closed as well as open treatment gave clinically acceptable results. In a similar comparison by Throckmorton and Ellis,[2] patients treated by open reduction initially had a faster rate of improvement of maximum interincisal opening (MIO) as well as excursion to the nonfractured side, but eventually results for both groups were the same regardless of the mode of treatment. Haug and Assael[3] also reported that there was no difference in MIO, lateral excursion, and protrusion in the two groups, but Yang and colleagues[4] found that patients treated by closed reduction had more condylar mobility.

Similar differences in the status of the posttreatment occlusion have also been described in the literature. Smets and colleagues[5] and Ellis and colleagues[6] reported more malocclusions in those patients treated by closed methods, whereas Haug and Assael[3] and Takenoshita and colleagues[7] found no difference. Likewise, Haug and Assael[3] found no difference in facial contour, but Yang and colleagues[4] reported less chin deviation when an open reduction was done.

The problem with most comparative studies that have been reported is that they are generally retrospective rather than prospective and that there is

Department of Oral and Maxillofacial Surgery, School of Dentistry, Virginia Commonwealth University, Richmond, VA, USA
E-mail address: dmlaskin@vcu.edu

Oral Maxillofacial Surg Clin N Am 21 (2009) 193–196
doi:10.1016/j.coms.2008.12.005

considerable variation in the patient selection and outcome criteria used as well as in the follow-up time. In such situations, a meta-analysis can sometimes be used to combine the information and reach more accurate conclusions. By analyzing a group of studies in this manner, the power of detecting an overall treatment effect increases, making it easier to find differences or similarities that may not be revealed by individual studies. Such a meta-analysis has been reported by Nussbaum and colleagues.[8] To be included in this study, the reports had to involve both closed and open treatment of only unilateral condylar process fractures, have at least a 6-month follow-up period, and include data on at least one of the following variables: MIO, lateral excursion and protrusion, facial symmetry, and posttreatment temporomandibular joint or masticatory muscle pain. Thirty-two articles were identified in which both closed and open treatment were compared and, of these, 13 met the inclusion criteria. The results showed that there was no difference in MIO, protrusion, or facial symmetry between the two groups, but those with an open reduction had greater excursion to the nonfractured side and those with closed treatment had more frequent temporomandibular joint or masticatory muscle pain.

In evaluating the results of any meta-analysis one has to consider the nature of the data available. In this analysis, only 1 of the 13 studies included was prospective. Also, there were considerable differences in the surgical protocols and materials used for fixation, as well as in the length of time that patients with closed treatment were kept in maxillomandibular fixation. Furthermore, findings about facial asymmetry and temporomandibular joint and masticatory muscle pain were based on subjective observations. Moreover, many patients were lost to long-term follow-up and not included in the results. Thus, the current literature in which the two methods were directly compared does not provide a conclusive answer to the question of whether, when given a choice, closed or open treatment of condylar process fractures gives better long-term results. Therefore, until better-designed comparative studies are available that will allow evidence-based decisions to be made, one can only look at individual case series for some guidance.

MANAGEMENT OF CONDYLAR PROCESS FRACTURES IN THE ADULT

Four factors need to be considered when choosing whether an adult patient should be treated by a closed or open method: (1) whether the fracture is unilateral or bilateral, (2) whether the patient is dentulous or edentulous, (3) whether the fragments are in contact with one another, and (4) whether there are other fractures in the mandible. Based on these considerations, closed treatment in the adult is indicated in the following situations: (1) when treating unilateral or bilateral fractures in dentulous or edentulous patients when the segments are still in contact, (2) when treating a unilateral fracture with dislocation of the condyle in the dentulous patient with a stable occlusion, and (3) when treating unilateral or bilateral intracapsular fractures. On the other hand, an open reduction should be done (1) when treating either dentulous or edentulous patients when there are unilateral or bilateral fractures without contact of the segments, (2) when treating patients who need a solid mandible to correct an associated midface fracture, or (3) when interference from the fractured condylar process prevents the occlusion from being reestablished.

Although the potential for developing an ankylosis is less in an adult patient with a fracture of the condylar process than in a child with such a fracture, an ankylosis is still a possibility. This raises the issue of how long patients receiving closed treatment should be kept in maxillomandibular fixation. Although traditionally it was advised to maintain such fixation for 4 to 6 weeks to allow proper healing, more recent studies have shown that 3 to 4 weeks are sufficient except in elderly or edentulous patients.[9]

MANAGEMENT OF CONDYLAR PROCESS FRACTURES IN THE CHILD (See also the article by Myall elsewhere in this issue)

For the management of fractures of the condylar process in the child, a number of considerations, in addition to those that determine treatment in the adult, make modifications necessary. First, there are anatomic differences. In a child, the condylar process is smaller and therefore fixation is more difficult. Moreover, because the cortex is thinner, intracapsular fractures are more likely to occur. The capsule is also less developed and therefore the fragments are less contained. As a result, children with condylar process fractures are more likely than adults with such fractures to develop ankylosis.

A second consideration is the fact that children have a greater osteogenic potential than adults and this leads to more rapid healing. Although this offers the advantage of shorter periods of immobilization, it also presents a disadvantage by increasing the potential for ankylosis, particularly with intracapsular fractures.

A third factor to be considered in children is their lack of cooperation. As a result, they may be resistant to having maxillomandibular fixation even though it is the indicated treatment. It also means that they may not be compliant with the postfixation jaw exercise regimens needed to avoid the development of an ankylosis.

Finally, there is the role of the condylar process in mandibular growth in children. This raises the question of whether anatomic realignment of the condylar process is a necessary condition for normal growth to occur. Studies have shown that perfect alignment is not essential because of the excellent remodeling potential in the child.[10,11] However, it is essential that segments be in contact.

When all of these factors are taken into consideration, a rational approach to the management of condylar process fractures in the child should be to use closed treatment whether the fractures are unilateral or bilateral, as long as the segments are in contact and there is no mechanical interference that prevents reestablishment of the occlusion. An open reduction should be done only when there is mechanical interference or there is no contact of the segments, which can result in shortening of the ramus and an anterior open bite in bilateral cases or a crossbite and facial asymmetry in unilateral cases. In all instances, it is important to inform the parents that, as a result of possible damage to the articular surface of the condyle by the trauma that caused the fracture, mandibular growth may be retarded and periodic clinical examinations and radiographs need to be done to monitor the situation and determine whether further treatment may eventually be necessary to correct any facial deformity.

As previously mentioned, because of the risk of ankylosis in the child, long periods of maxillomandibular fixation are contraindicated. Patients with intracapsular fractures should never be immobilized and they should immediately be placed on range-of-motion exercises. For other fractures, the younger the patient, the shorter the fixation period should be; generally, 10 to 14 days are sufficient.

DISCUSSION

Despite the publication of many case studies, not enough information is available to form the basis for decisions regarding the management of fractures of the condylar process. Thus, one still needs to rely on a careful consideration of the treatment objectives, the potential risks involved, and sound clinical judgment in making a final therapeutic decision.

There are certain areas, however, in which there does appear to be consensus. In the child, with few exceptions, closed treatment is preferable, fixation periods should be as short as possible, compliance with a vigorous postfixation exercise program is essential, and patients should have long-term follow-up for possible mandibular growth retardation. When there is contact of the segments, perfect realignment is not necessary because of the good remodeling potential of the child.

In the adult, it is important to restore ramus height by an open reduction to avoid an open bite or a crossbite and mandibular deviation when (1) there are bilateral fractures without contact of the segments, (2) there is a unilateral fracture in an edentulous patient, or (3) there is a unilateral fracture in a dentulous patient with an unstable occlusion. Open reduction is also necessary when there is a need to establish a stable mandibular base for the treatment of associated midface fractures or when there is mechanical interference with establishing a proper occlusion. There is still no agreement regarding the specific indications for closed treatment in the adult. However, as Luyk[12] has stated, "if the principle of using the simplest method to achieve optimum results is to be followed, the use of closed reduction of [condylar] fractures should be widely used."

REFERENCES

1. Steisch-Scholz M, Schmidt S, Eckardt A. Condylar motion after open and closed treatment of mandibular condylar fractures. J Oral Maxillofac Surg 2005;63:1304–9.
2. Throckmorton GS, Ellis E. Recovery of mandibular motion after closed and open treatment of unilateral mandibular condylar process fractures. J Oral Maxillofac Surg 2000;29:421–7.
3. Haug RH, Assael LA. Outcomes of open versus closed treatment of subcondylar fractures. J Oral Maxillofac Surg 2001;59:370–5.
4. Yang WL, Chen CT, Tsay PK, et al. Functional results of unilateral mandibular condylar process fractures after open and closed reduction. J Trauma 2002; 52:498–503.
5. Smets ML, Van Damme PA, Stoelinga PJ, et al. Nonsurgical treatment of condylar fractures in adults. J Craniomaxillofac Surg 2003;31:162–7.
6. Ellis E, Simon P, Throckmorton GS. Occlusal results after open or closed treatment of fractures of the mandibular condylar process. J Oral Maxillofac Surg 2000;58:260–8.
7. Takenoshita Y, Ishibashi H, Oka M. Comparison of functional recovery after nonsurgical and surgical

treatment of condylar fractures. J Oral Maxillofac Surg 1990;48:1191–5.

8. Nussbaum ML, Laskin DM, Best AM. Closed versus open reduction of mandibular condylar fractures in adults: a meta-analysis. J Oral Maxillofac Surg 2008;66:1087–92.

9. de Amaratunga NA. The relation of age to the immobilization period required for healing of mandible fractures. J Oral Maxillofac Surg 1987; 45:111–3.

10. Walker RV. Traumatic mandibular condylar fracture dislocations. Am J Surg 1960;100:850–63.

11. Boyne PJ. Osseous repair and mandibular growth after subcondylar fracture. J Oral Surg 1967;25: 300–9.

12. Luyk NH. Principles of management of fractures of the mandible. In: Peterson LJ, Indresano AT, Marciani RD, et al, editors, Principles of oral and maxillofacial surgery, Vol 1. Philadelphia: JB Lippincott; 1992. p. 407.

Management of Mandibular Fractures in Children

Robert W.T. Myall, BDS, MD, FDS, FRCD(C)[a,b,]*

KEYWORDS

- Fractures • Mandibular • Children
- Management • Outcomes

> *There are as many opinions as there are people: Each has his own correct way.*
> Terence (circa 190–159 BC): Phormio

There are many opinions about the management of mandibular fractures in children, but few articles in the evidence-based literature address the topic. This is not surprising because these fractures are rare and few surgeons see enough of them to prospectively study the initial injury, its treatment, and its subsequent effect on growth and function. To guide surgeons treating mandibular fractures in children, this article first reviews the growth of the mandible, describes how injury can affect such growth, and explains how to harness the process of growth to good effect. This information is important in making therapeutic decisions about the management of such injuries. The article then reviews the various opinions regarding diagnosis, treatment, and outcomes. Then, as a counterpoint, the author presents his own approach developed over 30 years as a pediatric oral and maxillofacial surgeon. For information beyond this overview, refer to the bibliography of comprehensive articles from the last 50 years.[1–6]

Children have an immense capacity for healing in the shortest possible time with a minimum of complications. The assistance that growth can give, coupled with the inherent ability of young bone, periosteum, and soft tissues to adapt to new situations, is quite different from that which we see in adults. A body of pertinent clinical oral and maxillofacial literature amplifies this point, starting in the late 50s with an article by MacLennan.[7] However, it wasn't until Rowe's[8] landmark article in 1969 that a well thought out approach to pediatric mandibular fractures surfaced. It still is a must-read for surgeons dealing with the young. Recently the concept of accurate primary repair has been applied to children, mainly at the urging of Posnick[1] and supported by other experienced surgeons. We can look forward to an expansion of these concepts with the appearance of new materials and data, as is already apparent in the debate about use of rigid versus resorbable plating systems. However, so far we are surrounded again by opinions, with little evidence-based fact.

Mandibular growth can be increased or decreased by trauma and its treatment. Thus, long-term follow-up with an orthodontist is the rule. This enables aberrations of growth to be intercepted and treated with appliance therapy or by a combination of orthodontics and surgery at an appropriate juncture. Even in the best of circumstances, imaging of the child's facial skeleton is difficult, and the use of CT with the patient under general anesthesia is often appropriate. This is especially true in condylar injuries in general and more specifically in the very young.

Child abuse has been on the rise, and injuries are often inflicted to the head and neck regions. When a child has either soft- or hard-tissue

[a] Oral & Maxillofacial Surgery, School of Dentistry, Oregon Health & Science University, 611 SW Campus Drive, Portland, OR 97239, USA
[b] School of Medicine, Oregon Health & Science University, Portland, OR, USA
* Oral & Maxillofacial Surgery, School of Dentistry, Oregon Health & Science University, 611 SW Campus Drive, Portland, OR 97239.
E-mail address: myallr@ohsu.edu

Oral Maxillofacial Surg Clin N Am 21 (2009) 197–201
doi:10.1016/j.coms.2008.12.007

injuries, and the parents' stories are inconsistent with the findings or they conflict with those given by other family members, the specter of child abuse should always be entertained and appropriate referral made.

GROWTH AND DEVELOPMENT

A review of the salient points of growth and development will help the reader understand why various techniques have evolved. As noted, mechanisms of growth can be disturbed by the initial injury or they can be harnessed to aid subsequent treatment. The nonsurgical treatment of condylar fractures is an example of the latter. Growth accelerates two times in a child's life: once around 9 years of age and the again at the onset of puberty. In both instances, the onset in girls predates that in boys. These growth spurts coincide with the loss of facial fat deposits, which can unmask latent facial asymmetries that might require therapeutic intervention.

A baby's mandible and lower lip are retrusive and the chin is virtually nonexistent. This can lead to the misconception of mandibular injury in babies subjected to trauma. The linear radiolucency at the symphysis, formed as a result of the two sides of the mandible developing independently, simulates a fracture and can also mislead the unwary. Fusion takes place toward the end of the first year.

The mandible houses many tooth buds and, as these teeth mature and erupt, there is a corresponding expansion of the mandible and development of the alveolus. The mandible itself is bodily displaced by the growth of the surrounding soft tissues, and it is in response to these changes that condylar growth occurs. The perignathic soft tissues impart a functional need that is reacted to by both the bone and the cartilage of the region. The latter view was proposed formally by Moss[9] in his functional matrix theory of growth and it has withstood the test of time.

Both endochondral and periosteal-endosteal activity are important elements of mandibular growth. Principal sites of the latter type of growth are the posterior surface of the ramus, the coronoid processes, and the alveolus. At the same time that bone is being deposited at the posterior edge of the ramus, resorption takes place at its anterior edge, thereby increasing the length of the mandibular body. There is little change in the anterior of the mandible, with the chin being almost inactive after the first months of life.

The morphology of the condyles in infants and toddlers is of interest because it influences the patterns of fracture seen in these age groups.

The condylar neck is thick and short, thus resisting fracture, while the head is highly vascular and vulnerable to crush injury. This also contributes to the difficulty of imaging the area using routine mandibular radiographic views. The short condylar neck is difficult to project away from the petrous portion of the temporal bone and so CT is the imaging modality of choice.

The position of the developing and partially erupted teeth within the jaws dictates where screws or wires can be placed. The tooth bud position is readily appreciated as a bluish bulge once the mucoperiosteum is elevated. The stage of root resorption of the deciduous teeth is significant when considering their use for anchorage of arch bars or eyelet wires. One should not rely entirely on the radiographic appearance of these teeth because they alternately loosen and tighten during exfoliation and may only be of use as occlusal stops.

The bone of children has a lower modulus of elasticity, a lower bending strength, and a lower mineral content that adult bone, which account for the different patterns of fracture. Commonly, the fracture initiates at the upper border of the mandible and then travels horizontally before reappearing at the lower border. The overlying periosteum in the child, compared to that in the adult, is much thicker, more vascular, more loosely attached to the underlying bone, and capable of more rapid callus formation. This results in the accelerated healing of pediatric fractures. One aspect of young bone also often overlooked is its varied structure. The bone of a newborn is quite different histologically from the bone of an older child, which in turn is different from that of a mature adult. This is the basis for the differential growth process that produces overall enlargement of the mandible and changes in its shape.

IMAGING

Imaging an awake traumatized child is difficult at the very least and perhaps impossible. Waiting 24 hours or so for the initial pain and shock to subside often pays dividends. The panoramic radiograph is the first step in all but the very young, when CT is the modality of choice. Chacon[10] pointed out that fractures of the condyle can easily be overlooked on a panoramic view and CT should be used when there is the slightest doubt. A call to the radiologist to discuss the need for sedation or anesthesia is always appreciated. Periapical and occlusal radiographs are helpful in defining fractures in the symphyseal region, where panoramic views lack definition.

As noted previously, pediatric fractures often track horizontally before emerging at the upper and lower borders. Hints of this phenomenon in the mixed dentition are suggested by misshapen tooth crypts, widened periodontal ligament spaces, and open contact points.

Fracture locations after the age of 10 assume a pattern similar to that in adults.[11]

TREATMENT

The aims of treatment are to obtain bony union, to normalize the occlusion, to restore normal form and function, and to avoid impediments to normal growth. Conventional wisdom tells us that to best fulfill these aims, the bony fragments must be accurately aligned. Efforts to ensure this alignment have led to complex methods of treatment, including open reduction. However, perfect alignment is not always necessary to ensure complete success. Children differ from adults in that the final result is determined not merely by the initial treatment but also by the effect that growth has on form and function over time. Minor malocclusions left during the deciduous or mixed dentition stages will be corrected by eruption of teeth and growth of the alveolus. Minor bony irregularities will likewise be improved by growth if normal function is maintained. The prevention of secondary deformities associated with derangement of growth demands long-term follow-up and appropriate intervention by the surgeon or orthodontist. It is important to maintain a perspective longer than the 6 to 8 weeks generally required in adults.

The treatment of mandibular injuries in children frequently necessitates multiple general anesthetics because taking impressions, placing hardware, and even removing sutures may not be possible in young children when they are awake. Early consultation among all clinicians involved in the child's care is important to allow for the development of an efficient, integrated treatment plan.

There are many types of fixation that can be applied to mandibular fractures, ranging from maxillomandibular fixation, to lingual splints, to various forms of rigid fixation. Moreover, in certain circumstances, no fixation at all is necessary. The speed with which fractures in children heal at various ages, the complexity of the fracture, the presence of concomitant injury, and the clinician's own experience with a variety of surgical approaches all factor into making the appropriate treatment choice. In the very young, 2 weeks of immobilization is sufficient and, up to the age of puberty, 3 or 4 weeks will suffice in most instances.[12]

There is unresolved debate about whether resorbable plates have a true advantage over their titanium counterparts and whether the later should be removed at the end of treatment. Again, opinion unsupported by facts rules the debate. Frank discussion with the family about the pros and cons of each method will help lead to the best solution. Eppley[13] and Bos[14] reviewed both sides of the issue in the clinical controversies section of the *Journal of Oral & Maxillofacial Surgery* in 2005.

There is a misconception that children are unable to accept having their jaws wired together. This is not so. With age-specific appropriate explanation, and with the help and concurrence of the parents, the child will generally acquiesce. Wiring often is the method of choice in the very young. In the deciduous and mixed dentition, carefully placed eyelet wires are usually more efficient than arch bars. However, when there are insufficient teeth, circummandibular wires and pyriform rim, nasal spine, and zygomatic buttress anchorage can be used to provide maxillomandibular fixation. Lingual splints have a place alongside plates when it is important to maintain jaw mobility, as in the case of condylar fractures associated with symphyseal or body fractures. The custom-made splint maintains the transverse dimension of the arch and prevents splaying of the angles, as may occur with bilateral condylar fractures.

Open or closed management of fractures of the mandibular condyle is the most hotly debated aspect of all mandibular fractures in children and resides in the fact that clinicians forget that both soft and hard tissues are involved in condylar fractures. There is ample experimental evidence from the animal studies of Walker[15] and Boyne[16] that fractured condyles have a remarkable recovery potential. Some years later, these findings were substantiated radiographically by studies in children by Gilhous-Moe[17] and Lund.[18] The latter is a prospective study that showed that the younger the child and the smaller the displacement, the greater the likelihood of successful remodeling in the face of early mobilization. Indeed, nearly 80% of Lund's patients did not acquire any asymmetry. Dahlstrom,[19] in a 15-year follow-up study of another group of children, showed no radiographic or functional deficits in those who sustained fractures between 3 and 11 years of age. However, in teenagers, the anatomical and functional restitution was not as good, although it infrequently gave rise to objective symptoms. Thoren[20] concluded that immediate mobilization, even when there was complete dislocation of the condylar process, resulted in a satisfactory long-term functional outcome with minimal asymmetry.

This evidence underscores the fact that the bony elements of a child's condyle can significantly remodel following fracture, but what about the traumatized soft tissues? Moss's[9] functional matrix theory tells us that the epignathic soft tissues govern the growth of the mandible. Placing a child immediately into maxillomandibular fixation for up to 2 weeks allows the traumatized soft tissue to heal with "short" scars rather than the longer ones that would be produced by continued mobilization. This has the effect of "anchoring" the functional matrix and consequently hindering growth and leading to asymmetry. Therefore, when some fixation is necessary, light training elastics rather than maxillomandibular fixation should be used and an active exercise program should be started as soon as the child can cooperate. Extended periods of maxillomandibular fixation can lead to ankylosis in children and should be avoided.

The malocclusion seen immediately postinjury in children with condylar process fractures is generally caused by muscle spasm, which dissipates over 3 or 4 days without the use of maxillomandibular fixation. Once the initial pain is gone, the child should be encouraged to eat a normal diet as soon as possible and to practice opening and closing the mouth in a straight line in front of a mirror. Light training elastics should be used when there is sustained deviation on opening or when there is a developing occlusal discrepancy. Long-term physical therapy may be needed when functional deficits linger.

The child's growth needs to be monitored until after the pubertal growth spurt and this is best accomplished with the help of an orthodontist. Occasionally, functional appliances or corrective jaw surgery may be necessary to maintain symmetry during the active growth period in the rare child showing asymmetric growth.

The final issue to be addressed is the role of open reduction in the management of condylar process fractures. Open reduction should be rarely employed and saved for when there is condylar displacement into the middle cranial fossa or when normal jaw movements are obstructed. Adolescents with condylar fractures do not have the same adaptive capabilities as those in the younger age groups. However, even though the radiographic appearance may be abnormal, function is usually within normal limits, as pointed out by Dahlstrom.[19] Dodson[21] convincingly summarizes the management and outcomes of condylar fractures in his 2005 article.

SUMMARY

Treatment of mandibular fractures in children requires an understanding of growth and those mechanisms that facilitate it. The processes of growth, along with the increased cellular activity in the tissues involved, lead to early healing with far fewer complications than seen in adults. With the exception of condylar process fractures, all forms of fixation can be used, with maxillomandibular fixation being preferred in the younger age group. Most condylar process fractures can be treated with minimal or no periods of fixation and with active exercise programs. Care should extend well beyond the acute injury and its immediate treatment and requires longitudinal monitoring of growth, symmetry, and temporomandibular joint function. This is most successfully done with the cooperation of an orthodontist. These approaches have evolved from a combination of opinion and the retrospective study of case series over the last 50 years and will no doubt be refined further with time.

REFERENCES

1. Posnick JC, Wells M, Pron GE. Pediatric facial fractures: evolving pattern of treatment. J Oral Maxillofac Surg 1993;51:836–44.
2. Myall R. Condylar injuries in children: what is different about them? In: Worthington P, Evans J, editors. Controversies in oral and maxillofacial surgery. Philadelphia: WB Saunders; 1993. p. 191–200.
3. Posnick J. Management of facial fractures in children and adolescents. Ann Plast Surg 1994;33:442–57.
4. Haug RH, Foss J. Maxillofacial injuries in the pediatric patient. Oral Surg Oral Med Oral Pathol Oral Radiol Endod 2000;90:126–34.
5. Myall RWT, Dawson KH, Egbert MA. Maxillofacial injuries in children. In: Fonseca RJ, editor. Oral and maxillofacial surgery, 3. Philadelphia: Saunders; 2000. p. 421–42.
6. Zimmermann CE, Trulis MJ, Kaban LB. Pediatric facial fractures: recent advances in prevention, diagnosis and management. Int J Oral Maxillofac Surg 2006;35:2–13.
7. MacLennan WD. Fractures of the mandible in children under the age of six years. Br J Plast Surg 1956;9:125–9.
8. Rowe N. Fractures of the jaws in children. J Oral Surg 1969;27:497–507.
9. Moss M, Salentijn L. The primary role of functional matrices in facial growth. Am J Orthod 1909;55:566–77.
10. Chacon GE, Dawson KH, Myall R, et al. A comparative study of 2 imaging techniques of the diagnosis of condylar fractures in children. J Oral Maxillofac Surg 2003;61(6):668–72.
11. Thoren H, Iizuka T, Halliikainen D, et al. Different patterns of mandibular fractures in children: An

analysis of 220 fractures in 157 patients. J Cranio-maxillofac Surg 1992;20:292–6.

12. Amaratunga N. The relation of age to the immobilization period required for healing of mandibular fractures. J Oral Maxillofac Surg 1987;45:111–3.

13. Eppley BL. Use of resorbable plates and screws in pediatric facial fractures. J Oral Maxillofac Surg 2005;63:385–91.

14. Bos RR. Treatment of pediatric facial fractures; the case for metallic fixation. J Oral Maxillofac Surg 2005;63:382–4.

15. Walker R. Traumatic mandibular condyle dislocations: effect on growth in the *Macaca* rhesus monkey. Am J Surg 1960;100:850–63.

16. Boyne P. Osseous repair and mandibular growth after subcondylar fractures. J Oral Maxillofac Surg 1967;25:300–9.

17. Gilhous-Moe O. Fractures of the condyle in the growth period. Stockholm: Scandinavian University Books; 1969.

18. Lund K. Mandibular growth and remodeling processes after condylar fracture. Acta Odontal Scand 1974;32(64):1–117.

19. Dahlstrom L, Kahnberg K-E, Lindahl L. Fifteen year follow-up on condylar fractures. Int J Oral Maxillofac Surg 1989;18:18–23.

20. Thoren H, Hallikainen D, Tateyuki L, et al. Condylar process fractures in children: a follow up study of fractures with total dislocation of the condyle from the glenoid fossa. J Oral Maxillofac Surg 2001;59(7):768–73.

21. Dodson TB. Condyle and ramus condyle unit fractures in growing patients: management and outcomes. Oral Maxillofac Surg Clin North Am 2005;17:447–53.

Management of Nasal Fractures

Vincent B. Ziccardi, DDS, MD*, Hani Braidy, DMD

KEYWORDS

- Nasal fractures • Nasal trauma • Nasal bone fractures
- Open reduction • Closed reduction

Because of the prominence of the nose and its central location on the face, nasal fractures are the most common facial fracture. They are estimated to occur in approximately 39% of patients with maxillofacial trauma.[1] The peak incidence of nasal fractures occurs in 15- to 30-year-olds, with a 2:1 male to female ratio. In this age group, altercations and sports injuries account for most nasal fractures, followed by falls and motor vehicle accidents. For the pediatric and geriatric group, most injuries are related to falls and accidents, with less sex predilection noted.[2]

Even though nasal fractures are the most frequently encountered facial fracture, controversies still exist regarding timing for repair, use of closed versus open techniques, and use of general versus local anesthesia for treatment. Before addressing these issues, however, it is important to know how to diagnosis nasal fractures.

DIAGNOSIS OF NASAL FRACTURES

The force required to fracture the nasal bones is less than that of other facial bones because of their prominent position and thinness. Strong forces from any direction can comminute the nasal bones, whereas fractures at the thicker root of the nose are often associated with concomitant facial fractures. With the intimate relationship of the skeletal and cartilaginous structures of the nose and septum, it would be unusual to see damage to one structure without damage to the others. Low velocity injuries usually result in septal fractures or dislocations along the vomerine groove, and high-velocity injuries often result in septal fractures through the thinner quadrangular cartilages. A fractured septum unfavorably affects the alignment of the nasal bones during healing and should be addressed during the management of nasal fractures.[3]

Epistaxis can occur with relatively minor nasal trauma because of the dense vascular network that supplies the nose known as Kiesselbach's plexus. Bleeding may also result from other areas of the nose, with anterior bleeding usually caused by the anterior ethmoidal artery, a branch of the ophthalmic artery, and posterior bleeding caused by a branch of the sphenopalatine artery.[4] The internal nasal structures are best visualized with a speculum examination after packing the nose with a vasoconstrictor for several minutes. All blood clots should be removed with saline irrigation and suction. Particular attention should be paid to the nasal septum for evidence of mucosal injury, perforation, or displacement. Mucosal lacerations may indicate an underlying nasal fracture. Understanding the mechanism of injury can be useful in the assessment of nasal fractures, in particular whether the vector of trauma was direct or from a lateral direction.

Plain radiographs generally are not helpful in the diagnosis of isolated nasal bone fractures, and they also do not provide imaging of the cartilaginous structures. Positive diagnosis of nasal bone fractures on such radiographs was reported to be only 82%, negative findings were 9.5%, and suspicion of fracture was 8.5% in a recent retrospective analysis of nasal bone fractures.[5] The authors concluded that computed tomography (CT) scanning is necessary because of the number of undiagnosed fractures with plain films alone. CT scanning is also indicated when there are associated facial injuries.

Department of Oral and Maxillofacial Surgery, University of Medicine and Dentistry of New Jersey, 110 Bergen Street, Room B-854, Newark, NJ 07103-2400, USA
* Corresponding author.
E-mail address: ziccarvb@umdnj.edu (V.B. Ziccardi).

Oral Maxillofacial Surg Clin N Am 21 (2009) 203–208
doi:10.1016/j.coms.2008.12.011

A thorough examination may be difficult in the presence of edema, ecchymosis, and dried blood or eschar. In these instances, it may be appropriate to re-evaluate the patient in several days, after the edema has resolved.[6] It is important to always rule out septal hematoma in all patients with nasal fractures. Failure to diagnose a septal hematoma can result in loss of septal cartilage and a saddle nose deformity, which will require more extensive reconstructive surgery. When a septal hematoma is identified, it should be evacuated and drained, along with use of appropriate splinting or packing to prevent re-accumulation of blood (**Fig. 1**).[7] The absence of a mucosal tear

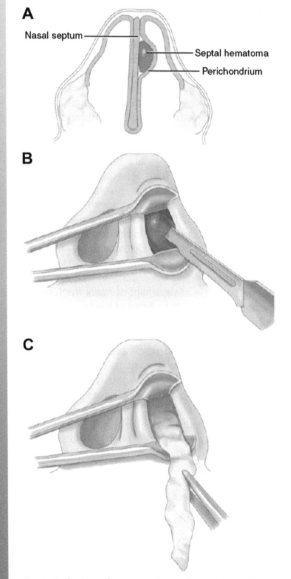

Fig. 1. Technique for evacuation of nasal hematoma. (*A*) Septal hematoma. (*B*) Incision and drainage of the hematoma. (*C*) Placement of drain.

or septal hematoma does not exclude septal damage. Septal injuries combined with nasal bone fractures are the major cause of nasal deformity and posttraumatic nasal obstruction.[8]

TIMING OF NASAL FRACTURE TREATMENT

There are differences of opinion regarding timing of the treatment of nasal fractures. If a patient is seen shortly after trauma, before significant edema develops, immediate treatment may be indicated. Other indications for immediate treatment include the presence of concomitant lacerations with exposure of the underlying skeletal or cartilaginous elements or the presence of a septal hematoma that requires immediate drainage. However, many surgeons opt to re-evaluate the patient in several days before performing definitive treatment. By re-evaluating a patient several days after the trauma, factors that may contribute to postoperative nasal deformity, such as acute edema, unrecognized pre-existing nasal deformity, and undetected septal fractures, can better be assessed before surgical intervention.[9]

Surgeons are aware of the difficulties encountered when attempting to correct nasal deformities after healing has occurred. Esthetic results are achieved more easily if full correction is performed early before significant scarring has taken place.[10] Patients who were able to undergo surgical management of their nasal fractures within the first 10 days of injury are less likely to require a revision septorhinoplasty. Outcomes of nasal fracture treatment may be compromised by the fact that late morphologic changes can occur over 1 or more years because of scarring.

LOCAL VERSUS GENERAL ANESTHESIA

Reduction of nasal fractures may be performed under local anesthesia supplemented with intravenous sedation or under general anesthesia. Fracture reduction under local anesthesia is an attractive alternative to general anesthesia because hospitalization and operating room utilization are not required, and it is a safe and efficient method to deal with these injuries. Studies comparing both techniques have determined there are no differences in clinical outcome as far as patient satisfaction.[11,12] Long-term satisfaction rates of more than 80% have been reported.[13] In the presence of minor nasal bony deviation and no associated septal or nasal tip displacement, closed reduction under local anesthesia has been suggested as the first line of treatment. Such a procedure is a safe, convenient and cost-effective

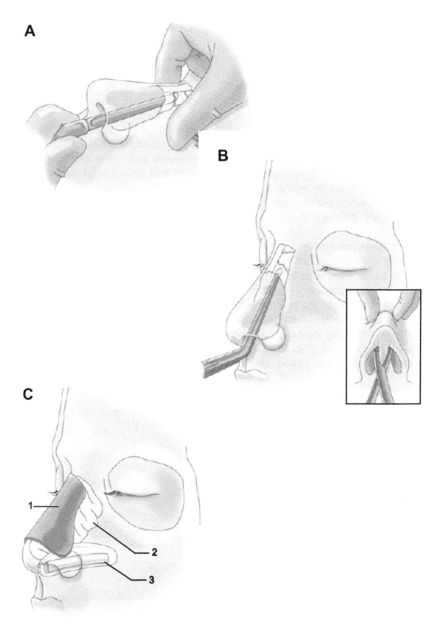

Fig. 2. Closed reduction of a nasal fracture. (*A*) Manipulation of nasal bones with elevator. (*B*) Septal reduction with Asch forceps. (*C*) Nasal packing and application of Denver splint.

method of treatment, with similar outcomes to general anesthesia in terms of postoperative pain and subsequent septorhinoplasty rates.[14] However, complex or severely displaced fractures may require treatment under general anesthesia. Moreover, secondary surgery, including rhinoplasty and septoplasty, has been reported to be required more often in patients having previously undergone closed reduction under local anesthesia compared with general anesthesia. Based on these facts, general anesthesia may be more effective than local anesthesia for the treatment of displaced

nasal fractures in that less subsequent corrective reconstructive surgery is required. It would appear that costs, potential risks, availability of facilities, severity of the injury, and surgeon preferences all contribute to the selection of local anesthesia versus general anesthesia in the management of nasal fractures.[15]

OPEN VERSUS CLOSED TECHNIQUES

Closed reduction is generally thought to be the simplest, safest, and easiest procedure to perform, with minimal potential morbidity. The decision to perform closed reduction rather than open reduction should be guided by the findings on clinical examination such as severity of the injury, degree of nasal obstruction, and amount of septal deviation and septal trauma. Comparison with a pretrauma photograph, when available, is often helpful in determining the amount of deformity. Closed reductions generally are a reasonable choice for most acute isolated nasal fractures with minimal bony and septal injury when performed within approximately 10 days of injury. Overall, closed reductions are performed with reasonable outcomes by different specialists with varied training.[16]

The objective of closed reduction is to reduce and align the skeletal and cartilaginous nasal structures to their pretrauma state and to maximize airway patency. Closed reduction is performed using an instrument such as an Asch forceps or blade handle placed internally to elevate the nasal bones, while externally molding the bony and soft tissues with the opposite hand (**Fig. 2**). Internal splints and packing are used based on the

surgeon's preference, and the nose is stabilized externally with a rigid splint. Internal packing, if used, is maintained for approximately 3 days, whereas external splinting is generally maintained for 7 to 10 days. A good airway and reasonable approximation of the pretrauma appearance often are obtainable goals (**Figs. 3** and **4**). However, this method of closed reduction may fail to adequately address deformities of the cartilaginous framework and nasal septum. It has been suggested that deviation of the nasal septum places stress on the nasal bones, causing them to displace after reduction.[17] The incidence of postreduction deformities after closed reduction that may require secondary rhinoplasty has been reported to range from 14% to 50%. Such revision surgery may be required for cosmetic reasons or for functional reasons, such as nasal obstruction. Therefore, preoperatively, it is essential to assess not only the nasal bone fractures but also the condition of the cartilaginous framework and septum before offering closed reduction to patients.[18] The final decision to perform open or closed reductions may be based on the condition of the septum and

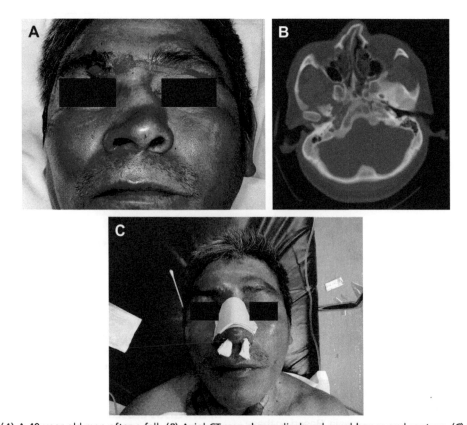

Fig. 3. (*A*) A 49-year-old man after a fall. (*B*) Axial CT scan shows displaced nasal bones and septum. (*C*) View of patient after closed reduction of nasal fractures under local anesthetic blocks in the emergency department and placement of nasal packing and a dorsal stent.

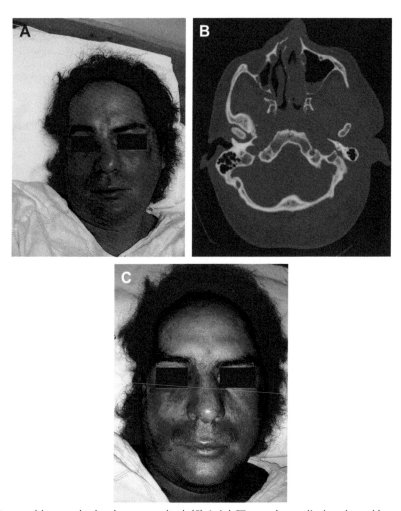

Fig. 4. (*A*) A 38-year-old man who has been assaulted. (*B*) Axial CT scan shows displaced nasal bones and septum. (*C*) View of patient immediately postreduction under local anesthesia in the emergency department before packing and placement of dorsal stent.

the need to preserve the connection between the septum, upper lateral cartilages, and nasal bones.[19] It has also been suggested that early full septorhinoplasty is indicated to avoid unfavorable outcomes from closed reduction because many patients will be reluctant to undergo a secondary procedure.

There is a lower rate of revision surgery in those patients who undergo open reduction of their nasal fracture with septoplasty as the initial treatment. If the cartilaginous septum cannot be reduced and replaced on the nasal crest of the maxilla by closed reduction, immediate septoplasty under general anesthesia to swing the septum into a more normal position is recommended.[20] It has been reported that patients with nasal fractures associated with septal deviation requiring septoplasty have fewer revision

septorhinoplasties performed if the initial procedure is an open surgical approach.

SUMMARY

The goal of treatment for nasal fractures is to restore the pretraumatic state and normal function. The decision by the surgeon regarding the surgical approach should be based on the degree of injury, the presence of concomitant facial injuries, patient compliance, training of the surgeon, and the presence and degree of septal injury. It should be understood clearly that the nasal bones follow the position of the septum. Although patients with an acute, isolated nasal injury and no significant septal involvement generally can be treated by closed reduction in the emergency department or outpatient clinic under local anesthesia, once the septum is involved, it is preferable to treat the patient in the operating room under general anesthesia to allow proper management of the septum. The use of a closed or open approach will then depend on the extent of the injury.

REFERENCES

1. Haug RH, Prather JL. The closed reduction of nasal fractures: an evaluation of two techniques. J Oral Maxillofac Surg 1991;49:1288–92.
2. Karagama YG, Newton JR, Clayton MGG. Are nasal fractures being referred appropriately from the accident and emergency department to ENT? Injury 2004;35:968–71.
3. Mondin V, Rinaldo A, Ferlita A. Management of nasal bone fractures. Am J Otol 2005;26:181–5.
4. Kucik CJ, Clenney T, Phelan J. Management of acute nasal fractures. Am Fam Physician 2004;70: 1315–20.
5. Hwang K, You SH, Kim SG, et al. Analysis of nasal bone fractures: a six year study of 503 patients. J Craniofac Surg 2006;17:261–4.
6. Ridder GJ, Boedeker CC, Fradis M, et al. Technique and timing for closed reduction of isolated nasal fractures: a retrospective study. Ear Nose Throat J 2002;81:49–54.
7. Cox AJ. Nasal fractures- the details. Facial Plast Surg 2000;16:87–94.
8. Rhee SC, Kim YK, Cha JH, et al. Septal fracture in simple nasal bone fracture. Plast Reconstr Surg 2004;113:45–52.
9. Rohrich RJ, Adams WP. Nasal fracture management: minimizing secondary nasal deformities. Plast Reconstr Surg 2000;106:266–73.
10. Fernandes SV. Nasal fractures: the taming of the shrewd. Laryngoscope 2004;114:587–92.
11. Owen GO, Parker AJ, Watson KF. Fracture-nose reduction under local anesthesia. Is it acceptable to the patient? Rhinology 1992;30:89–96.
12. Waldron J, Mitchell DB, Ford G. Reduction of fractured nasal bones: local versus general anaesthetic. Clin Otolaryngol 1989;14:357–9.
13. Wild DC, El Alami MA, Conboy PJ. Reduction of nasal fractures under local anaesthesia: an acceptable practice? Surg J R Coll Edinb Irel 2003;1:45–7.
14. Khwaja S, Pahade AV, Luff D, et al. Nasal fracture reduction: local versus general anaesthesia. Rhinology 2007;45:83–8.
15. Courtney MJ, Rajapakse Y, Duncan G, et al. Nasal fracture manipulation: a comparative study of general and local anesthesia techniques. Clin Otolaryngol 2003;28:472–4.
16. Staffel JG. Optimizing treatment of nasal fractures. Laryngoscope 2002;112:1709–19.
17. Green KMJ. Reduction of nasal fractures under local anaesthetic. Rhinology 2001;39:43–6.
18. Hung T, Chang W, Vlantis AC, et al. Patient satisfaction after closed reduction of nasal fractures. Arch Facial Plast Surg 2007;9:40–3.
19. Verwoerd CDA. Present day treatment of nasal fractures: closed versus open reduction. Facial Plast Surg 1992;8:220–3.
20. Fattahi T, Steinberg B, Fernandes R, et al. Repair of nasal complex fractures and the need for secondary septorhinoplasty. J Oral Maxillofac Surg 2006;64:1785–9.

Management of Orbital Fractures

Risto Kontio, MD, DDS, PhD[a],*, Christian Lindqvist, MD, DDS, PhD[a,b]

KEYWORDS

- Blow-out • Orbital surgery • Orbital reconstruction
- Fracture of orbit • Resorbable • Bone graft

Trauma to the orbital region can result in considerable facial deformity and can affect vision and the nervous system of the face. Rehabilitation of the patient requires an understanding of the alteration in form and function of the orbit, including the intraorbital and intraocular tissues, and the materials and methods available for repair.

The indications for surgery on orbital floor fractures are controversial. Strong indications include enophthalmos greater than 2 mm, significant hypoglobus, or diplopia. Certain consensus also prevails regarding the need for surgery when there is an increase of orbital volume more than 1 cm^3. When there are lesser degrees of trauma, disagreement remains regarding the best method of treatment.

The timing of surgery for orbital fractures has also been a controversial issue. Orbital fractures differ from all other facial fractures in that surgery does not typically attempt to achieve bone healing. Rather, the goal of surgery is simply to reconstruct the defect area of the fractured wall. As such, delaying the operation for varying periods of time is feasible. Rarely can it be considered an emergency operation.

The material of choice for wall reconstruction has also been under continued debate. There is general agreement that the ideal material for repairing the orbital floor should be rigid enough to support the orbital contents and should restore the original orbital form and volume. It should be safe and user friendly so that even inexperienced surgeons can handle it. It is the responsibility of the surgeon to recognize the diversity of the materials available and to apply them selectively in clinical use.

INDICATIONS FOR ORBITAL FRACTURE SURGERY

Several factors need to be considered in determining whether surgical intervention is indicated in a patient with an orbital fracture. A careful history and thorough physical examination are integral components in making decisions regarding the subsequent management of these patients.

There is general agreement that lack of ocular motility is an important consideration. Motility limitation can be graded on a scale from 0 to 4, where 0 equals no limitation (normal) and 4 equals no movement in the field of gaze. Each limited field of gaze represents a 25% reduction in motility. The most commonly accepted cause for limited motility is entrapment of the extraocular muscles (inferior rectus muscle) or their fascia into a fracture gap in the orbital floor.

Diplopia is another consideration. Although it may be a consequence of muscle entrapment, it can also result from muscle edema, hemorrhage in the orbital cavity, and motor nerve palsy. Another plausible cause is direct injury to the extraocular muscles or nerves. Diplopia correlates better with the severity of orbital injury than with the change of orbital volume.[1] Surgery may increase the risk of diplopia, at least temporarily.

Enophthalmos is another factor to consider and is usually a sign of a large orbital wall defect (**Fig. 1**A, B). Most practitioners define this as greater than 1 cm^3. The underlying cause of enophthalmos is a discrepancy between the volume of the orbital soft tissues and the bony orbital cavity. Enophthalmos greater than 2.0 mm typically indicates the need for surgical

^{a} Department of Oral and Maxillofacial Surgery, Helsinki University Hospital, 00029 HUS, Helsinki, Finland
^{b} Institute of Dentistry, University of Helsinki, POB 41, FIN-00014, Helsinki, Finland
* Corresponding author.
E-mail address: risto.kontio@hus.fi (R. Kontio).

Oral Maxillofacial Surg Clin N Am 21 (2009) 209–220
doi:10.1016/j.coms.2008.12.012

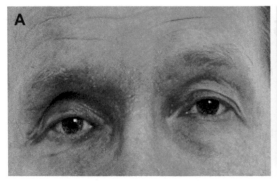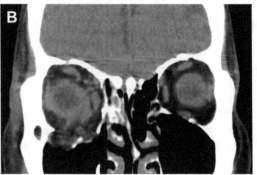

Fig. 1. (*A*) Patient with severe right enophthalmos and hypophthalmos after an injury in a basketball game. (*B*) Coronal CT scan showing the difference in orbital volume between the two sides.

intervention; however, factors such as globe tethering by entrapment, fat necrosis, and posterior soft tissue necrosis also may lead to enophthalmos. Furthermore, an orbital floor defect alone will not necessarily cause enophthalmos if the integrity of the fascial sling supporting the eye is intact.[2] Clinical judgment aided by CT imaging is crucial if operation is considered in patients with enophthalmos. Post injury edema and hemorrhage can cause the false illusion of proptosis and mask a true enophthalmos.

The ability to recognize enophthalmos is crucial for the surgeon. Ahn and coworkers recently published a study related to orbital volume change and late enophthalmos assessed by CT scanning.[3] There seems to be a direct relationship between the increase of orbital volume and measured enophthalmos. In cases with an orbital volume increase of less than 1 mL, the extent of enophthalmos is around 0.9 mm, whereas at a volume of 2.3 mL the enophthalmos is 2 mm. For every 1 mL increase of volume there is approximately a 0.9 mm increase in enophthalmos;[3] however, in normal orbits, there can be a natural volume difference of up to 8% between the left and right sides.[3]

TIMING OF ORBITAL SURGERY

The timing for orbital fracture repair is controversial. Proper surgical timing for an orbital fracture is paramount for producing good results. It has been suggested that there is an increase in complications such as adhesions and fibrosis with late or delayed surgery, which can lead to unsatisfactory outcomes; however, orbital fractures differ from all other facial fractures in that surgery does not typically attempt to achieve bone healing. The goal of surgery is simply to restore the preinjured form of the orbital walls. As such, delaying the operation for varying periods is often recommended. This delay is beneficial in

allowing the requisite orbital swelling to resolve, facilitating accurate diagnosis and strengthening the indications for surgery.

Rarely can orbital fracture repair be considered urgent; however, the ideal time to intervene after fracture occurrence cannot be precisely defined. Surgical timing differs in each case depending on the patient's age, fracture type (size, location, displacement, and comminution), functional impairment, esthetic deformities, and other clinical and radiographic findings. These factors should be weighed and individualized in each case. A classification system with treatment algorithms and timing of surgery exists for numerous other forms of maxillofacial trauma but not for orbital trauma.

Koorneef and Zonneveld[4] has suggested a conservative approach to blow-out fractures. In 1983, Hawes and Dortzbach,[5] and later Leitch and coworkers,[6] advocated surgery for orbital floor fractures within 14 and 21 days after trauma. On the other hand, Cole and coworkers[2] have suggested that urgent treatment should be considered in the case of traumatic optic neuropathy. Visual acuity and color desaturation testing must be performed if such an injury is suspected. The use of steroids and decompression has been suggested. Corticosteroids can be used as the only treatment if the visual acuity is better than 20/400.

Another indication for urgent surgery is an orbital fracture combined with an oculocardiac reflex.[7] The symptoms include a vagal tone response with bradycardia, heart block, nausea, vomiting and syncope. The change in vagal tone is presumable related to soft-tissue entrapment. The condition may be fatal; therefore, it should be managed with urgent surgical intervention. Urgent surgery is also indicated for orbital wall fractures in children associated with ocular motility limitations. The soft and flexible bones of children can result in a trap door fracture leading to entrapment of the soft tissues. A defect opens in the orbital floor and, because of the greenstick nature of the fracture, it subsequently closes leading to the entrapment. This phenomenon is sometimes called a "white-eyed appearance." Limitation of ocular motility should always lead to suspicion of possible muscle incarceration.[8]

Early surgery is inevitably required for penetrating craniocerebral injuries such as missile or nonmissile injuries associated with possible shock waves. Early surgery is also necessary when orbital wounds are caused by needles, scissors, knife blades, or other sharp objects. Presumed trivial orbital wounds may actually involve severe trauma, and these injuries should lead to a high index of suspicion related to penetrating craniocerebral injuries. CT scans with a bone window setting should be performed in all suspected cases not only to rule out the presence of a retained foreign body but also to define the site and extent of injury. High energy trauma with shock waves and cavity formation can result in severe complications including vascular injuries. In these patients, angiography should be considered. Early surgical intervention might decrease, among others things, the chance of formation of intracranial scar tissue and an epileptic focus. This possibility was suggested by Chibbaro and Tacconi,[9] who noticed that none of the patients who had early surgery developed epilepsy. The longest follow-up was 13 years.

De Man and coworkers[10] have suggested that young patients with severely restricted eyeball motility, an unequivocally positive forced duction test, and CT findings indicating a blow-out fracture of the orbital floor should undergo operative treatment as soon as possible after injury, whereas a wait and see policy, keeping the patient under observation, seems to be appropriate for blow-out fractures in adults. Matteini and coworkers and Grant and coworkers[7,11] found that in pediatric patients with diplopia, early repair resulted in more rapid improvement of symptoms than late treatment; they suggested that a symptomatic trap door fracture in young patients should be considered an indication for urgent treatment. In these studies, the timing of surgery for orbital fracture was strongly related to a combination of the following parameters: (1) the anatomic location of the fracture, (2) the presence of open or penetrating wounds, (3) the presence of cerebrospinal fluid leakage, (4) the patient's age, (5) functional impairment or muscle entrapment, and (6) serious forms of compression or ischemia.

MATERIALS FOR RECONSTRUCTION

Several different materials are available for restoration of the orbital walls, and there is no consensus about which is preferable; however, there is general consensus that the ideal material for orbital floor repair should be strong enough to support the orbital contents, inexpensive, readily available, easy to contour, resorbable, and, most importantly, biocompatible. One factor that has had a direct impact on the evolution of surgical management of internal orbital fractures is the increased availability of numerous biomaterials for reconstructing the bony contours and restoration of the proper orbital volume (**Tables 1** and **2**) (**Box 1**).

Autogenous Grafts

Autogenous tissues were among the first materials used to reconstruct the internal orbit and are still in frequent use today.[12–15] They involve a second operative site, which increases morbidity, and require a longer operative time to harvest. Some of these tissues are limited in quantity and are plagued by variable amounts of resorption over time.[16] Unpredictable resorption and the potential for late enophthalmos are the most critical arguments against the use of autogenous materials, particularly regarding autogenous bone grafts and, to a lesser degree, cartilage. Autogenous cartilage grafts are also too flexible to provide adequate support for the orbital contents when there are large defects.[17] Ilankovan and Jackson report that cartilage in its fresh state has a tendency to warp and is unsatisfactory for reconstruction of bony orbital walls.[18]

Autogenous bone grafting (**Fig. 2**A, B) has been the gold standard in providing a framework for repair of the injured facial skeleton and orbital walls.[12,14,19] The advantages of autogenous bone are its relatively good resistance to infection, its replacement by host bone through creeping substitution, the lack of a host response against the graft, and the lack of risk for late extrusion. Nevertheless, resorption and reduction of graft volume is a concern for long-term success.[16]

Basically there are two forms of nonvascularized autogenous bone grafts—cortical and cancellous. Cancellous grafts are revascularized more rapidly and more completely than are cortical grafts; however, cancellous bone imparts little mechanical strength. When cancellous bone is used to reconstruct large continuity defects, additional stabilization and rigid fixation, such as a titanium mesh system, are required.[20] A corticocancellous graft usually produces the best results by combining the attributes of both forms.[20]

Different sources such as calvarium, iliac crest, mandible, maxilla, and rib have been used.[12,21–24] Currently, calvarial bone seems to be the best choice for orbital wall reconstruction;[12,23]

Table 1
Advantages and disadvantages of autogenous, allogeneic, and xenograft materials for orbital wall reconstruction

Characteristic	Autogenous Grafts		Allogeneic Grafts			Xenografts	
	Bone	Cartilage	Bone	Dura	Fascia/Cartilage	Bone	Dermis
Resistance to infection, long term	FF	FF	F	F	F	F	U
Facilitates bone growth	FF	—	F	F	F	F	U
No foreign body reaction	FF	FF	F	F	F	UU	UU
Adequate mechanical properties	FF	U	FF	F	U	FF	UU
No second operative site	UU	UU	FF	FF	FF	FF	FF
No donor site morbidity	U	U	FF	FF	FF	FF	FF
Easy to harvest	F	F	FF	FF	FF	FF	FF
Easy to mold	U	F	U	F	F	U	F
Adequate in quantity	FF	F	FF	FF	FF	FF	FF
Low resorption	U	F	UU	F	F	UU	F
No risk of transmission of infectious agent	FF	FF	U	U	U	U	U

Abbreviations: FF, very favorable; F, favorable; U, unfavorable; UU, very unfavorable.

however, the anterior iliac crest is still the most common site.[25]

An autogenous bone graft from the anterior iliac crest is a favorable reconstruction material because enough bone is always available, and it can be harvested simultaneously with the orbital exploration; however, an iliac crest bone graft is bulky unless trimmed, and it may resorb unpredictably. Bartkowski and Krzystkowa and de Visscher and van der Wal used corticocancellous iliac crest bone for orbital floor or medial wall reconstruction in their follow-up studies and

Table 2
Advantages and disadvantages of alloplastic implant materials for orbital wall reconstruction

Characteristic	Nonresorbable Alloplastic Materials					Resorbable Alloplastic Materials				
	Tit	Sil	Tef	HA	BAG	PDS	PLLA	PLDLA	PGA	PLA/PGA
Resistance to infection	F	U	U	U	F	U	U	U	U	U
Facilitates bone growth	U	U	U	F	F	U	F	F	F	F
No foreign body reaction	F	U	U	F	F	U	U	U	U	U
Adequate mechanical properties	FF	F	F	F	FF	U	F	F	U	F
No second operative site	FF	FF	FF	FF	FF	FF	FF	FF	FF	FF
No donor site morbidity	FF	FF	FF	FF	FF	FF	FF	FF	FF	FF
Easy to harvest	FF	FF	FF	FF	FF	FF	FF	FF	FF	FF
Easy to mold	FF	FF	FF	F	U	F	F	F	F	F
Adequate in quantity	FF	FF	FF	FF	FF	FF	FF	FF	FF	FF
Low resorption	FF	FF	FF	F	FF	UU	F	F	UU	U
No risk of transmission of infectious agent	FF	FF	FF	FF	FF	FF	FF	FF	FF	FF

Abbreviations: BAG, bioactive glass; FF, very favorable; F, favorable; HA, hydroxyapatite; PDS, polydioxanone; PGA, polyglycolide; PLA/PGA, polylactide/polyglycolide; PLDLA, poly L/D lactide copolymer; PLLA, poly L lactide; Sil, silicone; Tef, Teflon; Tit, titanium; U, unfavorable; UU, very unfavorable.

Box 1
Different implant materials available for orbital wall reconstruction

Tissue grafts

Autogenous grafts (same individual)

    Bone

    Cartilage

    Dermis

    Dura mater

    Fascia

Allogeneic grafts (same species but separate genotype [allograft, homograft])

    Bone

    Cartilage

    Dermis

    Dura mater

    Fascia

Xenografts (another species)

    Biocoral

    Bone

    Dermis

Alloplastic materials

Nonresorbable nonmetal

    Bioactive glass

    Hydroxyapatite

    Polyethylene

    Silicone

    Teflon

Nonresorbable metal

    Titanium

    Vitallium

Resorbable

    Polydioxanone

    Polyglycolides

    Polylactides

bone is a rigid material, and the intraoperative three-dimensional assessment and accurate placement of such a bone graft is difficult. Although the resorption rate is high, this can be compensated by a slight overcorrection to allow for some of the remodeling. The rate of enophthalmos and hypophthalmos is low (**Fig. 4**).

Possible donor site problems with autogenous iliac bone grafts include nerve and blood vessel injuries, chronic pain, gait disturbances, and scar formation; however, considering the large number of autogenous iliac crest grafts used, the donor site morbidity seems to be low.[29,30] The results of a recent study are in accordance with these findings.[1] The main complication was the skin scar. It was recommended that the incision be carefully planned, especially in female patients, because 20% of patients end up having a visible scar in this area. Although the complication rate seems to be low, the donor site complications should not be ignored.[1]

Allogeneic Grafts

Allogeneic materials have been used successfully for orbital wall reconstruction; however, their use is decreasing because of concern over the antigenicity of the material and the potential transmission of infectious disease.[31]

Xenografts

Xenogeneic bone was popular in the 1960s but fell into disfavor due to reports of patients developing autoimmune diseases following bovine bone transplants.[32] In theory, the transmission of infectious disease is possible when xenografts are used, although no such reports are available in the literature.

Xenografts are rarely used for the repair of internal orbital fractures. Only a few case reports are available regarding their application within the orbit. A severe inflammatory reaction with a granulomatous component has been reported after the use of porcine dermis in orbital wall reconstruction.[33–35]

Alloplastic Materials

Alloplasts have gained popularity for reconstruction of the internal orbit because of their ease of use and the fact that there is no donor site morbidity. Other benefits of alloplasts include shorter operation times, the large variety of sizes and shapes available, and their seemingly endless supply. The alloplasts can be classified into those that are nonresorbable and those that are resorbable (see **Table 2**).

concluded that it was well tolerated and an adequate material for such repair.[26,27] Their results are similar to those of many other researchers.[12,16,23,28]

Kontio and coworkers[1] also found that reconstruction of the orbital walls with iliac bone was reliable, restoring the volume and the shape of the orbit well (**Fig. 3**A, B). Nevertheless, iliac

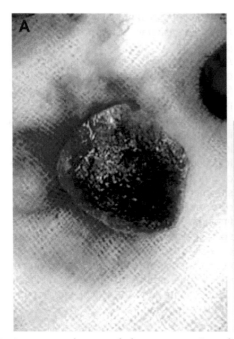
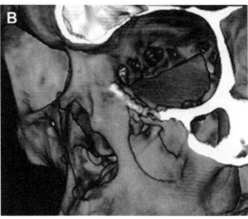

Fig. 2. Autogenous bone graft for reconstruction of the orbital floor. (*A*) Free iliac crest bone graft shaped to match the orbital floor. (*B*) CT three-dimensional view showing a free iliac bone graft in place to reconstruct fractured orbital floor.

Nonresorbable alloplasts

Nonresorbable alloplastic materials include titanium, silicone, polytetrafluoroethylene, polyethylene, hydroxyapatite, and bioactive glass. Titanium plates are thin, stiff, and easy to contour. They are easily stabilized, maintain their shape, and have the unique ability to compensate for volume without the potential for resorption. When titanium plates were introduced, it was generally believed that they did not need to be removed because titanium is a highly biocompatible material;[36] however, it has been shown that both titanium and aluminum are released from commercially pure titanium into adjacent areas and even into regional lymph nodes.[37,38] The clinical relevance of this release is not yet known. It has been suggested that in pediatric surgery, in areas of bony resorption and deposition, metallic plates should be removed due to plate displacement and restriction of growth.[39]

Further disadvantages of titanium implants in orbital wall reconstruction include extrusion due to dehiscence of the covering soft tissue and the risk of infection. There is also a theoretical risk of injury to the tissues of the orbital apex from a subsequent blow to the orbit. Because of the mesh structure, the orbital implant is difficult to remove.

Titanium implants have been used to span large defects in the internal orbit and provide a platform for bone graft support. This technique has proved to be reliable, and bone graft positioning is more secure. The infection rate has been reported to be 5%.[40] It was not until the reports by Sargent and Fulks and Sugar and coworkers that metals alone were routinely used for orbital reconstruction without an intervening bone graft or alloplast between the metal and the orbital soft tissues.[41,42] Many researchers have concluded that titanium mesh implants are a simple and reliable option for routine orbital floor repair.[12,42,43] Several types of titanium mesh plates are available (**Fig. 5**A, B).

Rubin and coworkers compared the use of custom-shaped orbital floor titanium plates with vitallium mesh and autogenous bone grafts.[44] They reported no significant complications related to the orbital implants. Metal implants were easier to use than autogenous bone grafts.

Silicones (polyorganosiloxanes) are synthetic polymers of silicon and oxygen (known as siloxane) modified with various organic groups attached to the silicon atoms. Silicone rubber is a chemically inert material available in block and sheet forms.

Polytetrafluoroethylene (Teflon) is a long-chain halogenated carbon polymer made by the polymerization of tetrafluoroethylene gas at high temperature and pressure. Both materials evoke a mild fibroblastic or inflammatory reaction.[45,46] Both have been used for orbital wall reconstruction even though they are not osteogenic, osteoconductive, or osteoinductive. Widely varying

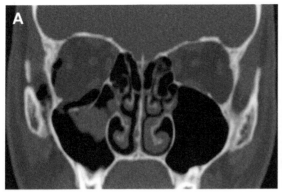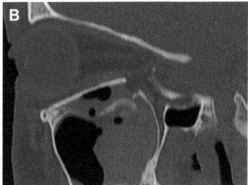

Fig. 3. (*A*) Coronal view of orbital floor after reconstruction with an iliac crest bone graft. (*B*) Sagittal view of patient. Note the good position of the graft.

complications have arisen from the use of these alloplastic implants, such as inferior eyelid swelling, pain, ocular dystopia, maxillary sinusitis, extrusion, and local infection.[47,48]

Porous polyethylene is a highly inert material. Its porous character allows for rapid fibrovascular and soft tissue ingrowth and eventual incorporation by bone. High-density porous polyethylene implants have been used successfully for correction of mild-to-moderate posttraumatic enophthalmos.[49] In a series of 140 patients, there was just one instance of implant infection requiring removal and no implant migration or exposure.[50] Other investigators also have concluded that porous polyethylene sheets offer advantages when used for orbital reconstruction.[51] They seem to permit predictable, stable results with few complications.

Hydroxyapatite has been used for both primary and secondary reconstruction of the orbital walls. Both hydroxyapatite block scaffolding and computer-aided machined hydroxyapatite ceramic implants have proved to be useful alternatives to metallic floor implants and autogenous bone grafts

in the reconstruction of large traumatic orbital floor defects.[52,53]

Bioactive glasses are silicates containing sodium, calcium, and phosphate as their main network modifier components. The chemical bonding of BAGs and bone has been demonstrated, and the materials have proved to be biocompatible and nontoxic.[54–56] Bioactive glass is osteoconductive in humans.[57] Studies have demonstrated that bioactive glass particles of a small size (300–355 μm [Biogran]) have the capacity to stimulate bone formation without contact with pre-existing bone.[58]

Good results have been achieved with this material in frontal sinus surgery.[59] However, only a few studies are available on the use of bioactive glass in orbital wall reconstruction. In a prospective study, Kinnunen and coworkers[60] compared the use of bioactive glass with conventional autogenous grafts (cartilage with or without lyophilized dura) for the repair of orbital floor defects after trauma. They concluded that bioactive glass was well tolerated and showed adequate maintenance of orbital and maxillary sinus volume without any evidence of resorption.

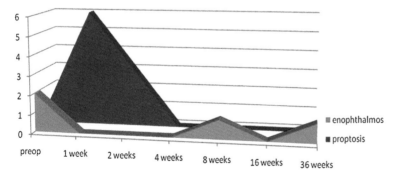

Fig. 4. Total number of patients with enophthalmos and proptosis of 2 mm or more during each clinical follow-up after iliac crest graft reconstruction. N = 24, prospective study. (*Adapted from* Kontio RK, Laine P, Salo A, et al. Reconstruction of internal orbital wall fracture with iliac crest free bone graft: clinical, computed tomography, and magnetic resonance imaging follow-up study. Plast Reconstr Surg 2006;118:1365–74; with permission.)

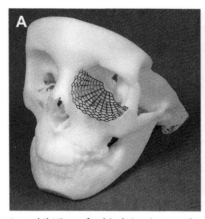
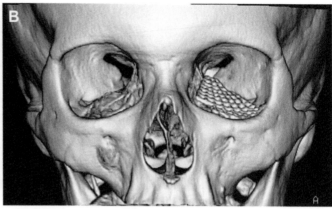

Fig. 5. (*A*) View of orbital titanium mesh plate 0.4 mm in thickness (Synthes) on a plastic skull model. (*B*) View of this type of plate being used for reconstruction of a large orbital wall defect.

Resorbable alloplasts

Biodegradable polymers (**Fig. 6**) have been used for biomedical applications for many years. Polyglycolide, polylactide, and polydioxanone (PDS) all degrade in vitro and in vivo by hydrolysis.[61] PDS has been mainly used for sutures, cords, pins, and screws in experimental and clinical orthopedic surgery.[62,63] It is usable in soft tissue, tendon, and ligament surgery because of its flexibility.[64] PDS has been reported to be well tolerated by the body and does not give rise to clinically detectable inflammatory reactions.[62]

New bone formation has been noted when PDS is used for orbital wall reconstruction.[65] It is easy to cut to suitable sizes, can be shaped and adjusted, and retains its structural integrity long enough for a sufficiently rigid scar to be formed.[65,66] Resorption occurs within 1 year. Because of resorption, overcorrection was thought to be necessary.[66] PDS is mechanically good enough for orbital reconstruction, and the overall results seem to be acceptable;[67] however, some studies have shown less favorable outcomes. The lack of osteoconductive properties was documented by Baumann and coworkers.[68] These investigators concluded that large defects in the orbital floor (more than 2.5 cm^2) cannot be reconstructed with a PDS sheet, which should be used only in cases without massive orbital fat herniation. These observations were similar to those in a study by Kontio and coworkers.[69] PDS did not act as an osteoconductive material, but bone healing took place in areas of displaced remnants of periosteum and bone fragments. In general, the fractured floor on the last postoperative CT scan was similar to that seen on the CT scan before operation.[69] It was concluded that floor reconstruction using PDS implants alone is inadequate. Merten and Luhr[70,71] and later de Roche and coworkers agreed with these results and further showed that PDS provokes adverse foreign body reactions. This phenomenon was confirmed in the study by Kontio and coworkers. MRI revealed adverse reactions in 63% of patients, thick scar formation in 38%, fibrotic sinuses filled with air or gas in 19%, and a fibrotic sinus with fluid formed around a PDS implant in 6% (**Fig. 7**). When the implants were removed, several small fragments of PDS were found inside a dense connective tissue capsule.[69]

Polylactide implants have been used for orbital floor reconstruction since 1972, when Cutright and Hunsuck published an experimental study on rhesus monkeys using 1.5-mm thick poly L lactide (PLLA) sheets.[72] They reported normal healing of the fracture and normal globe movements. The PLLA sheets were resorbed by phagocytes and giant cells with villous projections. Residual PLLA was detectable after 38 weeks, but no

Fig. 6. Resorbable implant (Synthes Polymax) for orbital wall reconstruction.

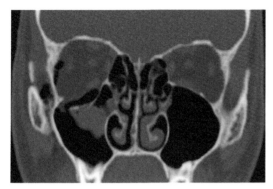

Fig. 7. CT scan at 4 month follow-up showing sinus involvement with a PDS orbital floor implant.

inflammatory reactions were seen. Similar findings were reported later by Rozema and coworkers.[73] In a study by Cordewener and coworkers,[74] the long-term outcome was evaluated after the repair of orbital floor defects with resorbable as-polymerized PLLA implants to determine whether these patients showed symptoms that could be indicative of the presence of a late tissue response. In the preceding years none of the patients had experienced any problems such as infection, migration, or extrusion of the implants, all of which might have indicated complications. The main drawback of PLLA implants is the low degradation rate and slow resorption in clinical use.[75]

The use of polyglycolide implants to treat 20 blow-out fractures has been reported.[76] Two patients complained of continuous infraorbital edema which, according to the investigators, was caused by poor residual drainage. The problem was resolved by regular massage of the region. Copolymers of biodegradable polyglycolide and polylactide acids have also been used for fracture treatment. Experimental studies have shown that this copolymer has a more rapid rate of degradation (9 to 15 months) than PLLA; therefore, it might be more suitable as an orbital implant material.[77] Clinical studies have shown good results with Lactosorb throughout the craniofacial skeleton.[78,79]

SUMMARY

Orbital surgery is not risk free. Complications include persistent pain and paresthesias, diplopia, and visual loss. The surgeon must always consider the potential complications against the possible benefits gained from the reconstruction procedure. Surgery is not always necessary. When there is small fracture, good ocular motility, and no significant enophthalmos or hypophthalmos, the surgeon should critically consider the risk/benefit

ratio. Reconstruction of the orbital walls with an iliac bone graft is a reliable procedure that restores the volume and shape of the orbit well; however, iliac bone is a rigid material, and the intraoperative three-dimensional assessment and accurate placement of the bone graft are difficult. The resorption rate is high, but most of it seems to be advantageous remodeling. Slight overcorrection is probably beneficial. No single factor can explain enophthalmos or hypophthalmos alone. Secondary operations seem to lead to a poor outcome. The question of which alloplastic material is most appropriate for reconstruction of the orbital walls remains unanswered.

REFERENCES

1. Kontio RK, Laine P, Salo A, et al. Reconstruction of internal orbital wall fracture with iliac crest free bone graft: clinical, computed tomography, and magnetic resonance imaging follow-up study. Plast Reconstr Surg 2006;118:1365–74.
2. Cole P, Boyd V, Banerji S, et al. Comprehensive management of orbital fractures. Plast Reconstr Surg 2007;120:57–61.
3. Ahn HB, Ryu WY, Yoo KW, et al. Prediction of enophthalmos by computer-based volume measurement of orbital fractures in a Korean population. Ophthal Plast Reconstr Surg 2008;1:36–9.
4. Koorneef L, Zonneveld FW. The role of direct multiplanar high resolution CT in the assessment and management of orbital trauma. Radiol Clin North Am 1987;4:753–9.
5. Hawes MJ, Dortzbach RK. Surgery on orbital floor fractures: influence of time of repair and fracture size. Ophthalmology 1983;90(9):1066–70.
6. Leitch RJ, Burke JP, Strachan IM. Orbital blowout fractures: the influence of age on surgical outcome. Acta Ophthalmol 1990;68:118–24.
7. Grant JH, Patrinely JR, Weiss AH, et al. Trapdoor fracture of the orbit in a pediatric population. Plast Reconstr Surg 2002;109:482–9.
8. Brannan PA, Kersten RC, Kulwin DR. Isolated medial orbital wall fractures with medial rectus muscle incarceration. Ophthal Plast Reconstr Surg 2006;3:178–83.
9. Chibbaro S, Tacconi L. Orbito-cranial injuries caused by penetrating non-missile foreign bodies. Acta Neurochir (Wien) 2006;148:937–42.
10. de Man K, Wijngaarde R, Hes J, et al. Influence of age on the management of blow-out fractures of the orbital floor. Int J Oral Maxillofac Surg 1991;20:330–6.
11. Matteini C, Renzi G, Becelli R, et al. Surgical timing in orbital fracture treatment: experience with 108 consecutive cases. J Craniofac Surg 2004;15:145–50.

12. Ellis E III, Tan Y. Assessment of internal orbital reconstruction for pure blowout fractures: cranial bone grafts versus titanium mesh. J Oral Maxillofac Surg 2003;61:442–53.

13. Converse JM, Smith B. Enophthalmos and diplopia in fractures of the orbital floor. Br J Plast Surg 1957;9:265–74.

14. Kaye BL. Orbital floor repair with antral wall bone grafts. Plast Reconstr Surg 1966;37:62–5.

15. Lai A, Gliklich RE, Rubin PA. Repair of orbital blowout fractures with nasoseptal cartilage. Laryngoscope 1998;108:645–50.

16. Sullivan PK, Rosenstein DA, Holmes RE, et al. Bonegraft reconstruction of the monkey orbital floor with iliac grafts and titanium mesh plates: a histometric study. Plast Reconstr Surg 1993;91:769–75.

17. Antonyshyn O, Gruss JS, Galbraith DJ, et al. Complex orbital fractures: a critical analysis of immediate bone graft reconstruction. Ann Plast Surg 1989;22:220–33.

18. Ilankovan V, Jackson IT. Experience in the use of calvarial bone grafts in orbital reconstruction. Br J Oral Maxillofac Surg 1992;30:92–4.

19. Marx RE. Clinical application of bone biology to mandibular and maxillary reconstruction. Clin Plast Surg 1994;21:377–92.

20. Tideman H, Samman N, Cheung LK. Functional reconstruction of the mandible: a modified titanium mesh system. Int J Oral Maxillofac Surg 1998;27:339–45.

21. Lee HH, Alcaraz N, Reino A, et al. Reconstruction of orbital floor fractures with maxillary bone. Arch Otolaryngol Head Neck Surg 1998;124:56–9.

22. Mintz SM, Ettinger A, Schmakel T, et al. Contralateral coronoid process bone grafts for orbital floor reconstruction: an anatomic and clinical study. J Oral Maxillofac Surg 1998;56:1140–4.

23. Dempf R, Gockeln R, Schierle HP. Autogene Knochentransplantate zur Versorgung der traumatisch geschädigten orbita. Ophthalmologe 2001;98: 178–84.

24. Siddique SA, Mathog RH. A comparison of parietal and iliac crest bone grafts for orbital reconstruction. J Oral Maxillofac Surg 2002;60:44–50.

25. St John TA, Vaccaro AR, Sah AP, et al. Physical and monetary costs associated with autogenous bone graft harvesting. Am J Orthop 2003;32: 18–23.

26. de Visscher JG, van der Wal KG. Medial orbital wall fracture with enophthalmos. J Craniomaxillofac Surg 1988;16:55–9.

27. Bartkowski SB, Krzystkowa KM. Blow-out fracture of the orbit: diagnostic and therapeutic considerations, and results in 90 patients treated. J Maxillofac Surg 1982;10:155–64.

28. Roncevic R, Malinger B. Experience with various procedures in the treatment of orbital floor fractures. J Maxillofac Surg 1981;9:81–4.

29. Banwart JC, Asher MA, Hassanein RS. Iliac crest bone graft harvest donor site morbidity: a statistical evaluation. Spine 1995;20:1055–60.

30. Ahlmann E, Patzakis M, Roidis N, et al. Comparison of anterior and posterior iliac crest bone grafts in terms of harvest-site morbidity and functional outcomes. J Bone Joint Surg Am 2002;84: 716–20.

31. Thadani V, Penar PL, Partington J, et al. Creutzfeldt-Jakob disease probably acquired from a cadaver dura mater graft: case report. J Neurosurg 1988; 69:766–9.

32. Pieron AP, Bigelow D, Hamonic M. Bone grafting with Boplant: results in thirty-three cases. J Bone Joint Surg Br 1968;50:364–8.

33. Converse JM, Smith B, Obear MF, et al. Orbital blowout fractures: a ten year survey. Plast Reconstr Surg 1967;39:20–3.

34. Morax S, Hurbli T, Smida R. Bovine heterologous bone graft in orbital surgery. Ann Chir Plast Esthet 1993;38:445–50.

35. Cheung D, Brown L, Sampath R. Localized inferior orbital fibrosis associated with porcine dermal collagen xenograft orbital floor implant. Ophthal Plast Reconstr Surg 2004;20:257–9.

36. Breme J, Steinhäuser E, Paulus G. Commercially pure titanium Steinhäuser plate screw system for maxillofacial surgery. Biomaterials 1988;9:310–3.

37. Moberg LE, Nordenram Å, Kjellman O. Metal release from plates used in jaw fracture treatment: a pilot study. Int J Oral Surg 1989;18:311–4.

38. Onodera K, Ooya K, Kawamura H. Titanium lymph node pigmentation in the reconstruction plate system of a mandibular bone defect. Oral Surg Oral Med Oral Pathol 1993;75:495–7.

39. Fearon JA, Munro IR, Bruce DA. Observations on the use of rigid fixation for craniofacial deformities in infants and young children. Plast Reconstr Surg 1995;954:634–7.

40. Glassman RD, Manson PN, Vanderkolk CA, et al. Rigid fixation of internal orbital fractures. Plast Reconstr Surg 1990;86:1103–9.

41. Sargent LA, Fulks KD. Reconstruction of internal orbital fractures with vitallium mesh. Plast Reconstr Surg 1991;88:31–8.

42. Sugar AW, Kuriakose M, Walshaw ND. Titanium mesh in orbital wall reconstruction. Int J Oral Maxillofac Surg 1992;21:140–4.

43. Mackenzie DJ, Arora B, Hansen J. Orbital floor repair with titanium mesh screen. J Craniomaxillofac Trauma 1999;5:9–16.

44. Rubin PA, Shore JW, Yaremchuck MJ. Complex orbital fracture repair using rigid fixation of the internal orbital skeleton. Ophthalmology 1992;99:553–7.

45. Lossing C, Hansson HA. Peptide growth factors and myofibroblasts in capsules around human breast implants. Plast Reconstr Surg 1993;91:1277–86.

46. Reno F, Lombardi F, Cannas M. UHMWPE oxidation increases granulocytes activation: a role in tissue response after prosthesis implant. Biomaterials 2003;24:2895–900.

47. Pauzie F, Cheynet F, Chossegros C, et al. Long-term complications of silicone implants used in the repair of fractures of the orbital floor. Rev Stomatol Chir Maxillofac 1997;98:109–15.

48. Rubin JP, Yaremchuk MJ. Complications and toxicities of implantable biomaterials used in facial reconstructive and aesthetic surgery: a comprehensive review of the literature. Plast Reconstr Surg 1997;100:1336–53.

49. Karesh JW, Horswell BB. Correction of late enophthalmos with polyethylene implant. J Craniomaxillofac Trauma 1996;2:18–23.

50. Romano JJ, Iliff NT, Manson PN. Use of Medpor porous polyethylene implants in 140 patients with facial fractures. J Craniofac Surg 1993;4:142–7.

51. Rubin PA, Bilyk JR, Shore JW. Orbital reconstruction using porous polyethylene sheets. Ophthalmology 1994;101:1697–708.

52. Ono I, Gunji H, Suda K, et al. Orbital reconstruction with hydroxyapatite ceramic implants. Scand J Plast Reconstr Surg Hand Surg 1994;28:193–8.

53. Lemke BN, Kikkawa DO. Repair of orbital floor fractures with hydroxyapatite block scaffolding. Ophthal Plast Reconstr Surg 1999;15:161–5.

54. Hench LL, Paschall HA. Direct chemical bond of bioactive glass-ceramic materials to bone and muscle. J Biomed Mater Res 1973;7:25–42.

55. Gross U, Strunz V. The interface of various glasses and glass ceramics with a bony implantation bed. J Biomed Mater Res 1985;19:251–71.

56. Aitasalo K, Kinnunen I, Palmgren J, et al. Repair of orbital floor fractures with bioactive glass implants. J Oral Maxillofac Surg 2001;59:1390–5.

57. Tadjoedin ES, de Lange GL, Holzmann PJ, et al. Histological observations on biopsies harvested following sinus floor elevation using a bioactive glass material of narrow size range. Clin Oral Implants Res 2000;11:334–44.

58. Huygh A, Schepers EJ, Barbier L, et al. Microchemical transformation of bioactive glass particles of narrow size range, a 0–24 months study. J Mater Sci Mater Med 2002;13:315–20.

59. Peltola M, Suonpaa J, Aitasalo K, et al. Obliteration of the frontal sinus cavity with bioactive glass. Head Neck 1998;20:315–9.

60. Kinnunen I, Aitasalo K, Pöllönen M, et al. Reconstruction of orbital floor fractures using bioactive glass. J Craniomaxillofac Surg 2000;28:229–34.

61. Williams DF. Review: biodegradation of surgical polymers. J Mater Sci 1982;17:1233–46.

62. Mäkelä P, Pohjonen T, Törmälä P, et al. Strength retention properties of self-reinforced poly L-lactide (SR-PLLA) sutures compared with polyglyconate (Maxon) and polydioxanone (PDS) sutures: an in vitro study. Biomaterials 2002;23:2587–92.

63. Plaga BR, Royster RM, Donigian AM, et al. Fixation of osteochondral fractures in rabbit knees: a comparison of Kirschner wires, fibrin sealant, and polydioxanone pins. J Bone Joint Surg Br 1992;74:292–6.

64. Vainionpää S, Rokkanen P, Törmälä P. Surgical applications of biodegradable polymers in human tissues. Progr Polym Sci 1989;14:679–716.

65. Cantaloube D, Rives JM, Bauby F, et al. Use of a cup-shaped implant of polydioxanone in orbital-malar fractures. Rev Stomatol Chir Maxillofac 1989;90:48–51.

66. Iizuka T, Mikkonen P, Paukku P, et al. Reconstruction of orbital floor with polydioxanone plates. Int J Oral Maxillofac Surg 1991;20:83–7.

67. Jank S, Emshoff R, Schuchter B, et al. Orbital floor reconstruction with flexible Ethisorb patches: a retrospective long-term follow-up study. Oral Surg Oral Med Oral Pathol Oral Radiol Endod 2003;95:16–22.

68. Baumann A, Burggasser G, Gauss N, et al. Orbital floor reconstruction with an alloplastic resorbable polydioxanone sheet. Int J Oral Maxillofac Surg 2002;31:367–73.

69. Kontio R, Suuronen R, Salonen O, et al. Effectiveness of operative treatment of internal orbital wall fracture with polydioxanone implants. Int J Oral Maxillofac Surg 2001;30:278–85.

70. Merten HA, Luhr HG. Resorbable synthetics (PDS foils) for bridging extensive orbital wall defects in an animal experiment comparison. Fortschr Kiefer Gesichtschir 1994;39:186–90.

71. de Roche R, Adolphs N, Kuhn A, et al. Reconstruction of the orbits with polylactate implants: animal experimental results after 12 months and clinical prospects. Mund Kiefer Gesichtschir 2001;5:49–56.

72. Cutright DE, Hunsuck EE. The repair of fractures of the orbital floor using biodegradable polylactic acid. Oral Surg 1972;33:28–34.

73. Rozema FR, Bos RR, Pennings AJ, et al. Poly(L-lactide) implants in repair of defects of the orbital floor: an animal study. J Oral Maxillofac Surg 1990;48:1305–9.

74. Cordewener FW, Bos RR, Rozema FR, et al. Poly(L-lactide) implants for repair of human orbital floor defects: clinical and magnetic resonance imaging evaluation of long-term results. J Oral Maxillofac Surg 1996;54:9–13.

75. Suuronen R, Pohjonen T, Hietanen J, et al. A 5-year in vitro and in vivo study of the biodegradation of polylactide plates. J Oral Maxillofac Surg 1998;56:604–14.

76. Sasserath C, Van Reck J, Gitani J. The use of a polyglycolic acid membrane in the reconstruction of the orbital floor and in loss of bone substance in the

maxillofacial region. Acta Stomatol Belg 1991;88:
5–11.

77. Wiltfang J, Merten HA, Becker HJ, et al. The resorbable miniplate system Lactosorb in a growing cranio-osteoplasty animal model. J Craniomaxillofac Surg 1999;27:207–10.

78. Ahn DK, Sims CD, Randolph MA, et al. Craniofacial skeletal fixation using biodegradable plates and cyanoacrylate glue. Plast Reconstr Surg 1997;99:1508–15.

79. Enislidis G, Pichorner S, Kainberger F, et al. Lactosorb panel and screws for repair of large orbital floor defects. J Craniomaxillofac Surg 1997;25:316–21.

Management of Naso-Orbital-Ethmoidal Fractures

Harry Papadopoulos, DDS, MD[a,b],*, Nader K. Salib, DDS[a]

KEYWORDS

- Naso-orbital-ethmoidal fractures
- Management • Controversies

Naso-orbital-ethmoidal (NOE) fractures remain the most complex of all facial fractures to diagnose and treat mainly because of the intricate anatomy and difficulty in fracture fixation. As the incidence of high-speed, high-force accidents has increased over the decades, so too has the number of such fractures. Due to the degree of force and the vectors involved, NOE fractures rarely occur as isolated events. Associated injures often include central nervous system injury, cribriform plate fracture, cerebrospinal fluid rhinorrhea, and fractures of the frontal bone, orbital floor, and middle third of the face, as well as injury to the lacrimal system.

Successful management of NOE fractures demands consideration of both the hard and soft tissues, as well as a comprehensive understanding the regional anatomy. Misdiagnosis and inadequate or delayed treatment often result in facial deformities and functional defects that are at best only partially correctable with secondary care.[1–4] As with the care for other types of maxillofacial fractures, clinicians continue to disagree about what treatment is best for NOE fractures. This article discusses these controversies and offers recommendations for therapy consistent with modern principles of maxillofacial trauma management.

CLINICAL DIAGNOSIS OF NASO-ORBITAL-ETHMOIDAL FRACTURES

Blunt trauma to the midface should always arouse suspicion of a potential NOE fracture. Such fractures are characterized by a short and retruded nasal bridge, telecanthus, enophthalmos, and a shortened palpebral fissure.[1,5–7] The combination of a thorough clinical examination and proper imaging delineates and confirms the extent of injury.

The initial evaluation consists of visual examination of the nasoethmoidal region. The general physical appearance varies with the extent of injury. NOE fractures associated with panfacial injuries are associated with a diffuse facial edema, whereas isolated NOE fractures are associated with localized ecchymosis and edema in the nasal and periorbital regions (**Fig. 1**A, B).[8]

Following the initial inspection, palpation of the regional structures should be performed using the bimanual nasoethmoidal examination.[9] The bimanual examination not only confirms the diagnosis of a questionable fracture but also determines the need for surgical repair.[8,9] First, using the index finger and thumb, the nasal bridge should be palpated for crepitation and bony movement. Next, a Kelly clamp is placed intranasally against the portion of the medial orbital rim directly opposite the medial canthal ligament. The index finger is then placed externally deeply over the medial canthal insertion. One should be sure that the examining finger is directly over the canthal ligament and not over the lateral aspect of the nose, as improper placement can result in misdiagnosis.[8,9] The examiner then tests for stability by assessing movement of the canthus-bearing

[a] Division of Oral & Maxillofacial Surgery, Department of Oral Surgery & Hospital Dentistry, Indiana University, 1050 Wishard Blvd., RG 4201, Indianapolis, IN 46202, USA
[b] Oral & Maxillofacial Surgery Residency Training Program, Indiana University, 1050 Wishard Blvd., RG 4201, Indianapolis, IN 46202, USA
* Corresponding author. Division of Oral & Maxillofacial Surgery, Department of Oral Surgery & Hospital Dentistry, Indiana University, 1050 Wishard Blvd., RG 4201, Indianapolis, IN 46202.
E-mail address: hp4@iupui.edu (H. Papadopoulos).

Oral Maxillofacial Surg Clin N Am 21 (2009) 221–225
doi:10.1016/j.coms.2008.12.008
1042-3699/08/$ – see front matter © 2009 Elsevier Inc. All rights reserved.

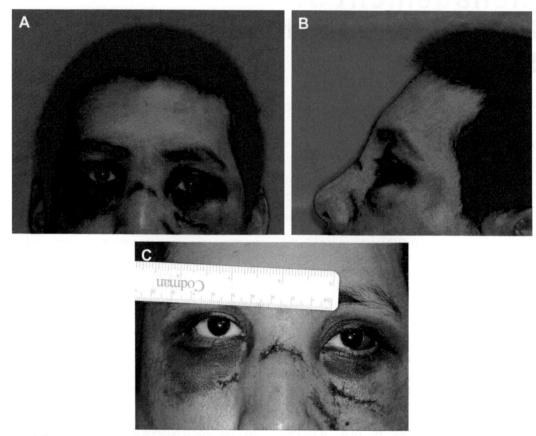

Fig.1. (*A*) Patient with NOE fracture. Note periorbital ecchymosis and edema. (*B*) Same patient. Note loss of nasal projection. (*C*) Same patient. Note telecanthus.

bone between the Kelly clamp placed against the medial orbital rim and the finger. Movement of the central fragment indicates instability of the fracture, requiring reduction and fixation. If no movement of the canthus-bearing segment is appreciated, operative repair is not needed. Non-displaced fractures with periorbital continuity also may not need operative reduction if fracture stability is confirmed during bimanual examination. However, displaced, impacted fractures, despite a lack of mobility, require treatment. When properly performed, the bimanual examination is the gold standard for physical examination of NOE fractures.

Disruption of the medial canthal ligament results in traumatic telecanthus. The average intercanthal distance is 33 to 34 mm for Caucasian males and 32 to 34 mm for Caucasian females.[5] Intercanthal distances greater than 35 mm are suggestive of a displaced NOE fracture, while those greater than 40 mm are diagnostic of such a fracture (**Fig. 1**C).[5] Medial canthal ligamental injury may be bilateral or unilateral. As such, the distance from each medial canthus to the nasal dorsum

should be noted and compared. Localized edema can distort the local anatomy and make accurate determination of the intercanthal distance impossible.[1] However, the intercanthal distance can be approximated, as it is approximately half of the interpupillary distance.

CONTROVERSIES IN THE MANAGEMENT OF NASO-ORBITAL-ETHMOIDAL FRACTURES

Before 1960, the treatment of NOE fractures generally involved closed reduction with external plates and splint fixation techniques.[1,6,10] The most important advancement in the treatment of such fractures came in 1964, when both Mustarde and Dingman[11,12] demonstrated superior results with open reduction and internal fixation using interfragmental wiring. Later, in 1970, Stranc[13] highlighted the incidence of the medial canthal tendon avulsion and advocated exploration through existing lacerations or local incisions and treatment with anterior transnasal wires. Current treatment modalities both combine and extend these previous contributions.

Early Versus Late Management

Although there is no absolute consensus in the literature as to how long one should wait before treating these fractures, some investigators have suggested waiting no more than 2 weeks.[1] Waiting longer increases the likelihood of requiring osteotomies to properly reduce and fix the fractures. Delayed repair is particularly difficult for type III injuries, which involve the canthal ligaments. Once healing and scarring have begun, finding the avulsed medial canthal ligament becomes more difficult. Also, scarring may prevent adequate correction of the intercanthal distance, even with proper reduction of the bones.[8] Therefore, one should treat these fractures as soon as possible. Treatment should begin as soon as the edema from the initial traumatic event has resolved, but waiting no later than 10 to 14 days, as long as the patient is stable enough to undergo the procedure.

Closed Versus Open Reduction

Proper management of the medial canthal tendon and the adjacent bones is the lynchpin to obtaining optimal results with NOE fractures. Closed reduction methods performed in the past, including those involving the use of external splints, have yielded poor esthetic results. Such techniques do not allow for the proper reduction of the medial canthal-bearing segment, leading to posttreatment telecanthus. Closed techniques also do not afford the opportunity to reestablish nasal projection, leading to posttreatment nasal deformities. Therefore, open techniques are now recognized as the best way to manage NOE fractures.

Management is generally dictated by the extent of injury, and this is best summarized by the Markowitz and colleagues[2] classification of NOE fractures. Type I injuries, where the medial canthal tendon is attached to a large fragment of bone, are the easiest to manage with three-point stabilization using rigid fixation at the nasofrontal junction, infraorbital rim, and piriform rim (**Fig. 2**A, B). Type II injuries show more comminution, yet still maintain an attached medial canthal tendon to a sizable bony fragment. Type III injuries show extensive comminution, with attachment of the medial canthal tendon to a small bony fragment or avulsion of the medial canthal tendon. Type II and type III injuries are managed in a similar fashion. For both types of injuries, fixation of the bony fragments is accomplished with a combination of microplates for larger bony segments and wires (28 or 30 gauge) for smaller bony segments. Location of the medial canthal tendon is necessary if it is attached to a small bony fragment or avulsed, either from the traumatic injury or inadvertent detachment by the surgeon. If direct visualization is difficult, grasping some of the tissues in the area of the tendon with forceps and pulling medially can aid in locating it. Once the medial canthal tendon is located, a wire is passed through the bony fragment in anticipation of the transnasal canthopexy. However, with tiny fragments, it can sometimes be difficult to secure a wire through this segment. Therefore, this situation is treated like an avulsion and a permanent suture is secured through the tendon. The other end of the suture is then tied to a wire. The wire then can be passed through the nasal bones using either an awl or a spinal needle to perform the transnasal canthopexy. The wire is then twisted while gently pulling it laterally, decreasing the intercanthal distance. It is also preferable to secure the wire on the contralateral side to a microplate or screw. Care should also be taken to ensure that there is no lateral flaring of the posterior aspect of the fracture as this will result in incomplete correction of the traumatic telecanthus. Therefore, the tendon is always suspended posterior and superior to its original location to overcorrect the intercanthal distance. Esthetically, an overcorrected result is far superior to an undercorrected telecanthus. Although difficult, "flipping" the coronal flap back and forth between the surgical sites while

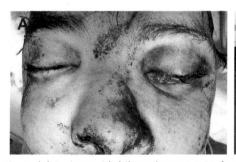
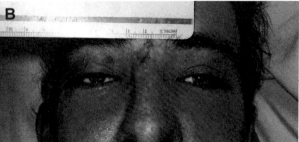

Fig. 2. (*A*) Patient with bilateral type I NOE fracture, preoperative view. (*B*) Same patient, postoperative view. Note corrected telecanthus.

measuring the intercanthal distance ensures an adequate correction of the traumatic telecanthus.

Surgical Access for the Treatment of Naso-Orbital-Ethmoidal Fractures

Various surgical approaches have been described for accessing NOE fractures. However, the coronal incision remains the gold standard. Careful release of the supraorbital and supratrochlear neurovascular bundles provides excellent access to the nasofrontal suture region as well as to the medial orbital walls. The coronal incision also allows access to the parietal bone for harvesting the dorsal strut graft. Other approaches, including the Lynch incision (**Fig. 3**) and open sky approach, although they may appear more direct, are actually more limited for access and result in scarring. Similarly, when patients have lacerations in the area, they frequently need to be extended to get adequate access, resulting in poor esthetics.

The midfacial degloving approach has also been described in the literature for the management of NOE fractures.[14] This approach has the advantage of avoiding any facial or scalp incisions. The author has never used this approach for NOE fractures. However, one can envision the difficulty in gaining access to the orbital floor and medial orbital wall with this approach.

Other approaches used in combination with the coronal incision include the transconjunctival or subciliary incision for access to the infraorbital rim and orbital floor, and a maxillary vestibular incision (intraoral) for accessing the piriform rim.

These adjunctive incisions also yield excellent cosmetic results. Once again, as with any maxillofacial fracture, wide access with exposure of all fractures is the rule. This allows the surgeon to visualize the reduction in three dimensions at multiple points.

Performing a Dacryocystorhinostomy at the Time of Fracture Treatment

Lacrimal dysfunction has not been noted to be a significant problem with NOE fractures unless treatment is delayed or performed secondarily.[15,16] Interestingly, an increased incidence of lacrimal dysfunction has been shown with closed techniques compared with open approaches.[13,17] Unless an obvious injury is noted, such as a laceration in the region of the nasolacrimal apparatus, routine exploration of the apparatus or a dacryocystorhinostomy is not indicated. A dacryocystorhinostomy should not be performed prophylactically as the incidence of nasolacrimal dysfunction after NOE injury is only 5% to 17.4%.[18]

Grafting the Nasal Dorsum

Type II and III injuries require reconstruction of the nasal dorsum with a bone graft to reestablish nasal projection. This is necessary for various reasons, including the loss of support from a weakened septum, comminution of the bones in the area, and prevention of a saddle nose.[1,3,4,8,17] Often, type III fractures also require reconstruction of the medial orbital wall with a bone graft.[1,3] This provides a stable strut of bone for reattachment of the medial canthal tendon and prevents enophthalmos. With the coronal flap elevated, a split thickness graft from the adjacent parietal

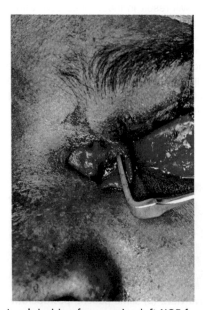

Fig. 3. Lynch incision for accessing left NOE fracture.

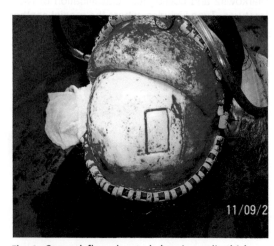

Fig. 4. Coronal flap elevated showing split thickness calvarium bone harvest.

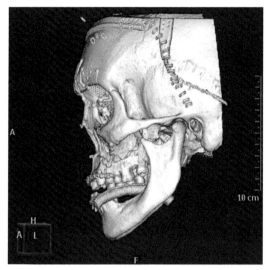

Fig. 5. Extension of nasal splint into naso-orbital soft tissue valley.

calvarium can easily be harvested to accomplish this (**Fig. 4**) and to reconstruct any orbital wall defects. Unless contraindicated, calvarium is the graft of choice. Other autogenous sites include the rib, ilium, and mandible.[3] When reestablishing nasal projection, the graft is secured to stable bone in the nasofrontal region with screws (**Fig. 5**). Alloplastic materials potentially increase the likelihood of infection and generally should be avoided.

SUMMARY

Management of NOE fractures requires an understanding of the local anatomy, a thorough clinical examination, and proper treatment planning. To achieve good results, one must emphasize early treatment, wide exposure through esthetic incisions, and reconstruction using rigid fixation and bone grafting where appropriate. Although managing these fractures can be extremely challenging, the results can be extremely gratifying.

REFERENCES

1. Ellis E III. Sequencing treatment for naso-orbito-ethmoid fractures. J Oral Maxillofac Surg 1993;51: 543–58.
2. Markowitz BL, Manson PN, Sargent L, et al. Management of the medial canthal tendon in nasoethmoid orbital fractures: the importance of the central fragment in classification and treatment. Plast Reconstr Surg 1991;87:843.
3. Herford AS, Ying T, Brown B. Outcomes of severely comminuted nasoorbitoethmoid fractures. J Oral Maxillofac Surg 2005;63:1266.
4. Gruss JS. Complex nasoethmoid-orbital and midfacial fractures: role of craniofacial surgical techniques and immediate bone grafting. Ann Plast Surg 1986; 17:377.
5. Paskert JP, Mason PN, Iliff NT. Nasoethmoidal and orbital fractures. Clin Plast Surg 1988;15:209.
6. McIndoe AH. Diagnosis and treatment of injuries of the middle third of the face. Braz Dent J 1941; 71:235.
7. Pecaro B, Erickson M. Naso-orbital ethmoidal fractures. Oral Maxillofac Surg Clin North Am 1990;2: 145.
8. Leipziger JS, Manson PN. Nasoethmoid orbital fractures. Current concepts and management principles. Clin Plast Surg 1992;19:219.
9. Paskert JP, Manson PN. The bimanual examination for assessing instability in naso-orbitoethmoidal injuries. Plast Reconstr Surg 1989;83:165.
10. Blair VP, Brown, Hamm WG. Surgery of the inner canthus and related structures. Am J Ophthalmol 1932;15:498.
11. Mustarde JC. Epicanthus and telecanthus. Int Ophthalmol Clin 1964;4:359–76.
12. Dingman RO, Grabb WC, Oneal RM. Management of injuries of the naso-orbital complex. Arch Surg 1969;98:566–71.
13. Stranc MF. Primary treatment of naso-ethmoid injuries with increased intercanthal distance. Br J Plast Surg 1970;23:8.
14. Cultrara A, Turk JB, Gady HE. Midfacial degloving approach for repair of naso-orbital-ethmoid and midfacial fractures. Arch Facial Plast Surg 2004;6: 133–5.
15. Merkx MA, Freihofer HP, Borstlap WA, et al. Effectiveness of primary correction of traumatic telecanthus. Int J Oral Maxillofac Surg 1995;24:344–7.
16. Becelli R, Renzi G, Mannino G, et al. Posttraumatic obstruction of lacrimal pathways: a retrospective analysis of 58 consecutive nasoorbitoethmoid fractures. J Craniofac Surg 2004;15:29–33.
17. Gruss JS, MacKinnon SE, Kassel EE, et al. The role of primary bone grafting in complex craniomaxillofacial trauma. Plast Reconstr Surg 1985;75:17.
18. Gruss JS, Hurwitz JJ, Nik NA, et al. The pattern and incidence of nasolacrimal injury in naso-orbital-ethmoid fractures: the role of delayed assessment and dacryocystorhinostomy. Br J Plast Surg 1985; 38:116.

Management of Frontal Sinus Fractures

R. Bryan Bell, DDS, MD, FACS[a,b,c]

KEYWORDS

- Frontal sinus • Cranio-maxillofacial • Surgery
- Trauma • Facial • Fractures • Skull base
- Nasal • Orbital • Ethmoidal

The goals in the treatment of frontal sinus injuries are to provide an esthetic outcome, restore function, and prevent complications. However, there is no consensus as to how to best achieve these goals. Unfortunately, the questions that Stanley[1] proposed in 1989 still lack definitive answers more than 19 years later: (1) Which fractures, if left untreated, will lead to an immediate or delayed complication? and (2) What is the appropriate surgical procedure if treatment of the fracture is deemed necessary? This article discusses the controversies in the surgical treatment of such fractures and provides a scientific rationale for proper management.

SURGICAL MANAGEMENT OF FRONTAL SINUS FRACTURES

Modern concepts regarding the management of the traumatized frontal sinus began in 1898 when Reidel[2] first described exenteration of the frontal sinus by completely removing the anterior and posterior tables along with the associated sinus mucosa. For many decades, various modifications of the exenteration (ablation) procedure remained the standard of care for complex fractures.[3–10] Beginning in the 1970s and largely in the pre-CT scan era, a handful of publications written by relatively few authors describing treatment in select patients, greatly influenced the management of frontal sinus injuries in the United States[1,11–30] More recent improvements in diagnostic imaging and surgical technology have now led to a wide variety of new philosophies, protocols, and procedures related to the treatment of frontal sinus injuries, each with the goal of providing an esthetic outcome, restoring function, and preventing complications.[31–40] These techniques principally include repair (open reduction and internal fixation of the anterior table), obliteration (ablation), and cranialization. An optimal strategy for the management of frontal sinus injuries, however, remains enigmatic, and indeed there is no consensus on when surgical intervention is indicated.

Classification

A number of classification schemes have been advocated by different investigators in an attempt to describe injury patterns for frontal sinus fractures and to provide a clinically relevant decision-making tool.[1,16–26,31–34] While a few fairly describe the various injury patterns, based on the intraoperative and radiographic examinations, most are too complicated to be clinically useful. The preferred classification scheme is that described by Raveh[41] in 1992 (**Fig. 1**). In it, the frontal, maxillary, and ethmoidal sinuses; the orbital cavity; and the nasal buttress are regarded as shock absorbers, trauma to which results in two broad injury categories: type I, which consists of fronto-naso-ethmoidal and medial orbital frame fractures without skull-base involvement; and type II, which consists of combined skull-base, fronto-naso-ethmoidal, and medial orbital frame fractures with frequent optic nerve compression.

---

[a] Oral and Maxillofacial Surgery Service, Legacy Emanuel Hospital and Health Center, 2801 N. Gantenbein, Portland, OR 97227, USA
[b] Department of Oral and Maxillofacial Surgery, Oregon Health & Science University, Mailcode: SDOMS, 611 SW Campus Drive, Portland, OR 97239, USA
[c] Head and Neck Surgical Associates, 1849 NW Kearney, Suite 300, Portland, OR 97209, USA
E-mail address: bellb@hnsa1.com

Oral Maxillofacial Surg Clin N Am 21 (2009) 227–242
doi:10.1016/j.coms.2008.12.003
1042-3699/08/$ – see front matter © 2009 Elsevier Inc. All rights reserved.

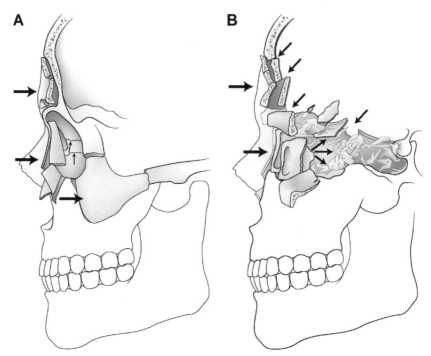

Fig.1. Classification of fronto-naso-orbital/skull-base fractures. (*A*) Type I. The external facial frame and buttresses give way and absorb and neutralize the impact, thereby preserving the posterior wall of the frontal sinuses, the frontal skull base, and the optic nerve canal. (*B*) Type II. These injuries are caused by high-energy forces that are not absorbed and neutralized by the external frame, and result in severe disruption of not only the external frame but also the internal palisades and buttresses.

In type I fractures, the external facial frame and buttresses give way and absorb and neutralize the impact, thereby preserving the posterior wall of the frontal sinus, the frontal skull base, and the optic nerve canal. These injuries are not characterized by significant brain injury or dural laceration, and are generally managed by reduction of the external frame fractures and the naso-orbital-ethmoidal component, if present. Type II fractures, on the other hand, are caused by high-energy forces that are not absorbed and neutralized by the external frame, and result in severe disruption of not only the external frame but also the internal palisades and buttresses. Type II fractures are characterized by intracranial dislocation of the posterior frontal sinus wall, inward telescoping of the nasal pyramid, and intracranial dislocations along the anterior skull-base planes, including the orbital roof and sphenoidal-parasellar areas. Significant neurologic injury is not uncommon, including dural tears, cerebrospinal fluid (CSF) leak, brain tissue herniation, intracranial hematoma, and optic nerve compression. Treatment often includes a subcranial or transcranial approach to remove (cranialize) the frontal sinus, repair underlying dural lacerations, and, if indicated, decompress the optic nerve.

Repair

Repair of the frontal sinus implies the preservation of the sinus anatomy, including the nasofrontal duct, sinus mucosa, and its anterior and posterior bony walls (**Fig. 2**). The fractures are approached via a standard coronal incision, or alternatively through existing lacerations if access is adequate. When raising the coronal flap, it is wise to also develop a robust pericranial flap that can be available as a potential obliteration material, if needed, or to line the anterior skull base and assist with dural repair, when necessary. Repair of any associated nasal or naso-orbital-ethmoidal fractures should be performed simultaneously, with care to properly restore nasal projection and nasofrontal contour.

Some investigators have advocated removal of the sinus membrane whenever it has been violated.[33] This is not a necessary step and, in our practice, no effort is made to remove the sinus membrane as long as nasofrontal drainage remains intact. Generally, the anterior table is anatomically reduced and then stabilized with titanium or resorbable plates and screws. Resorbable plates and screws are ideal for use in the cranium/frontal bone because they are nonfunctional bones without significant load.[42]

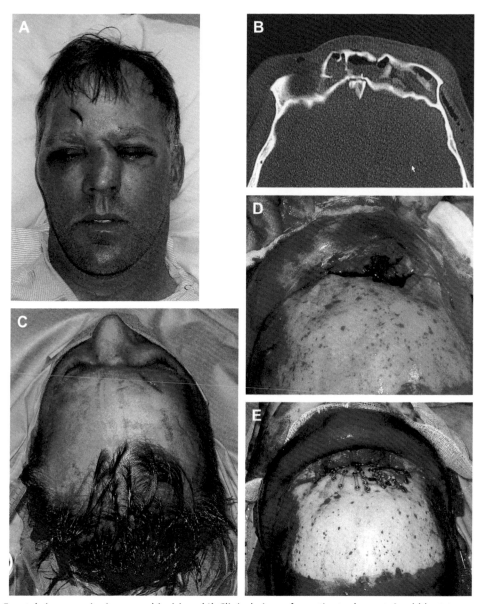

Fig. 2. Frontal sinus repair via coronal incision. (*A*) Clinical view of a patient who sustained blunt trauma from a motor vehicle accident and a Raveh type I fracture. Note displaced fronto-naso-orbital component. (*B*) Axial CT scan showing a displaced anterior table frontal sinus fracture. These types of injuries are amenable to repair of the anterior table alone, without removal of the sinus membrane or obliteration of the sinus. (*C*) Presurgical view of the patient prepared for a coronal approach. Male-pattern baldness is a consideration and the incision is placed more posteriorly than usual to conceal the scar within the hairline. (*D*) Surgical exposure via a coronal incision exposing the entire forehead and frontonasal complex. (*E*) Open reduction and internal fixation of the anterior table, in addition to repair of the naso-orbital-ethmoid fractures, using titanium plates and screws. (*F*) Frontal view of the patient 6 months postoperatively. (*G*) Profile view of the patient 6 months postoperatively.

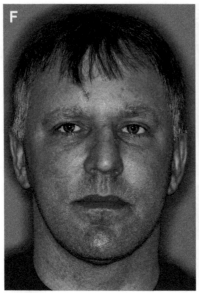 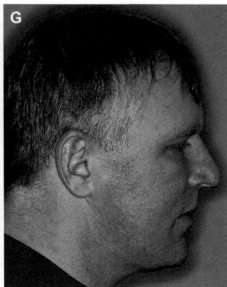

Fig. 2. (*continued*)

Endoscopic-Assisted Repair

Several investigators have reported cases in which anterior wall fractures of the frontal sinus have been treated using endoscopic techniques.[43–52] Some investigators have described simple reduction of the fractures, some performed open reduction and internal fixation of the fractures, and others camouflaged the anterior wall depression by endoscopically applying an alloplastic filler or implant.

The preferred technique allows for accurate reduction of the fractures combined with internal fixation using titanium mesh plates (**Fig. 3**). To date, this technique has been successful in five consecutive patients with isolated anterior wall defects and no evidence of nasofrontal duct obstruction. All patients were restored to form and function and there have been no complications. The technique used is similar to that for the endoscopic forehead lift, with one central and one or two lateral hairline incisions. The soft tissues are elevated in a subperiosteal plane and the fractures are visualized by means of a 30° endoscope with an external sheath for soft tissue retraction. Then, a stab incision is made in the eyebrow and skin hooks and endoscopic elevators are used to reduce the fragments. Once reduced, the fragments are stabilized with a titanium mesh plate inserted through the hairline incision. Screws are then placed through the brow stab incision.

Obliteration

Obliteration involves the elimination of the frontal sinus cavity while maintaining the anterior and posterior tables. The most important principles for successful obliteration include the meticulous removal of all visible mucosa, the removal of the inner cortex of the sinus wall, and the permanent occlusion of the frontonasal duct. The frontal sinus is treated as an isolated cavity, precluding any potential mucosal regrowth from the nasal epithelium.

The osteoplastic operation is generally performed though a coronal incision, but on occasion may be performed via existing forehead lacerations (**Figs. 4 and 5**). Care must be taken to place the incision well into the hairline for individuals experiencing alopecia or male-pattern baldness. In bald or balding men, alternative incisions, such as the "gull wing" or "open sky" incision, or other forehead approaches, can be used. In general, however, these incisions result in very poor esthetics and their use is highly discouraged. Dissection of the coronal incision is performed in a subgaleal plane and care is taken to develop a robust, anteriorly based pericranial flap for lining the anterior skull base or plugging the nasofrontal duct. The extent of the frontal sinus is estimated by direct examination or "sounding" of the sinus walls with an instrument. The anterior table is completely removed, exposing the underlying sinus cavity and allowing unimpeded access to all aspects of the sinus walls. The mucosal lining of the frontal sinus and the intersinus septum are removed using a rotating burr under loupe magnification or a surgical microscope. The frontonasal duct or recess is occluded using the pedicled pericranial flap, which is rotated into the sinus. The rest of the sinus is packed with autologous fat or other autologous or alloplastic material (see following section).

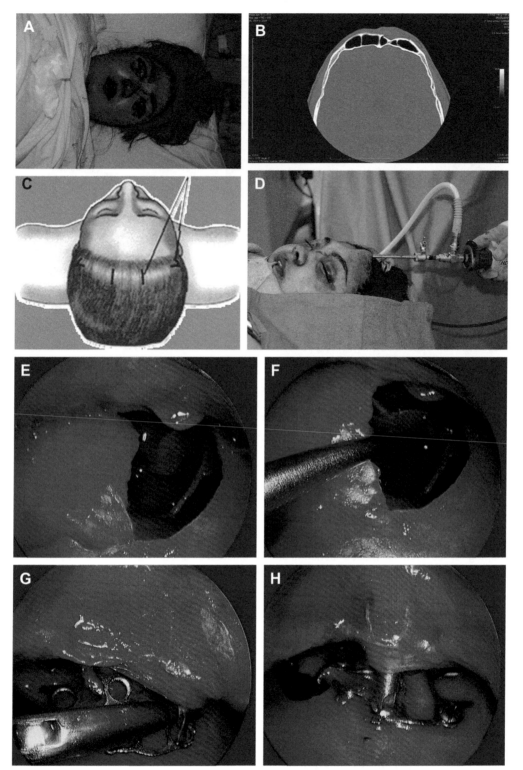

Fig. 3. Endoscopic-assisted frontal sinus repair. (*A*) View of 17-year-old female involved in a motor vehicle accident causing an isolated anterior table frontal sinus fracture without nasofrontal duct obstruction and an orbital blowout fracture. (*B*) Axial CT scan. (*C*) Incisions for endoscopic-assisted frontal sinus surgery. (*D*) Intraoperative view. (*E*) Endoscopic view of depressed anterior table frontal sinus fracture. (*F*) Endoscopic view showing reduction of the fractures using a skin hook. (*G*) Endoscopic view showing insertion of the titanium mesh plate. (*H*) Endoscopic view of plate fixation with the screwdriver inserted via a brow stab incision. (*I*) Endoscopic view of the fixed fracture. (*J*) Postoperative frontal view of the patient. (*K*) Postoperative submental view of patient. (*L*) Postoperative axial CT scan of the patient.

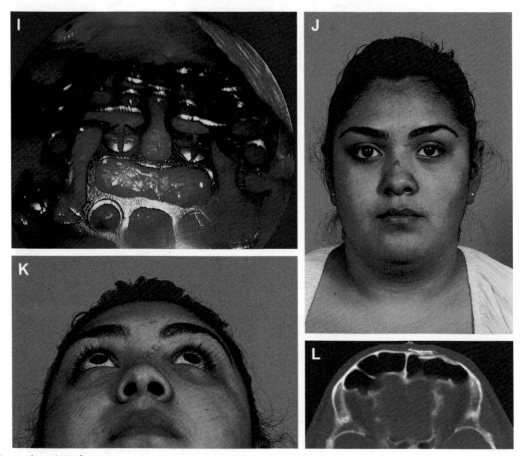

Fig. 3. (*continued*)

Special attention should be paid to the patient with telescoping or severely displaced concomitant frontonasal or naso-orbital-ethmoidal fractures. The nasal dorsum should be anatomically reduced from above, along with the anterior wall of the frontal sinus/frontal bone. The nasofrontal complex is then stabilized with titanium miniplates or bioresorbable plates and screws (see **Figs. 4** and **5**). Dorsal onlay bone grafting is rarely needed if the nasal bones can be anatomically reduced. The decision to repair, obliterate, or cranialize the sinus is often made intraoperatively, based on the extent of nasofrontal duct obstruction found during the procedure.

Biomaterials for Frontal Sinus Obliteration

A number of autogenous and alloplastic materials are available for use as filler in frontal sinus obliteration.[53] The volume of material needed is highly variable, averaging approximately 35 to 40 cm,[3] but with as much as 200 cm^3 needed in some cases. Although each material has its own advantages and disadvantages, autogenous grafts are preferable to allogeneic materials because of their extensive clinical history and favorable long-term treatment results.

Autogenous fat

Autogenous fat is currently the most widely used and well-suited material for frontal sinus obliteration.[4,8,54,55] The advantages of fat grafts include ease of harvest, minimal donor site morbidity, ample available volume, and favorable handling characteristics. The disadvantages lie primarily in the need for a donor site. Histologic studies have demonstrated predictable graft viability with prominent nuclei and vascular ingrowth.[56] Clinically, fat meets the anatomic and physiologic requirement for sinus obliteration by maintaining a barrier between the nasal cavity and neurocranium, thus preventing retrograde flow of microbes.

Autogenous muscle

Unpedicled temporalis muscle has been advocated by various neurosurgeons as a source of autogenous material for sinus obliteration.[9,55,57] It has the

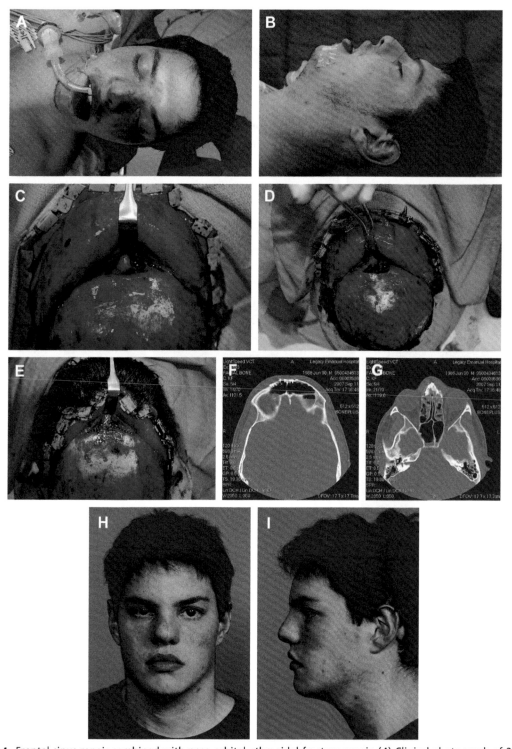

Fig. 4. Frontal sinus repair combined with naso-orbital-ethmoidal fracture repair. (*A*) Clinical photograph of 23-year-old male involved in a motor vehicle collision. (*B*) Profile view showing a telescoping, displaced naso-orbital-ethmoidal fracture. (*C*) Surgical exposure via coronal incision. (*D*) Reduction of nasal bone and nasofrontal region. Note that there is no nasofrontal duct obstruction. (*E*) Stabilization and fixation with titanium plates and screws. (*F*) Postoperative axial CT scan showing well-reduced anterior table. (*G*) Postoperative axial CT scan showing well-reduced naso-orbital-ethmoid fracture. (*H*) Postoperative facial appearance. (*I*) Postoperative profile view.

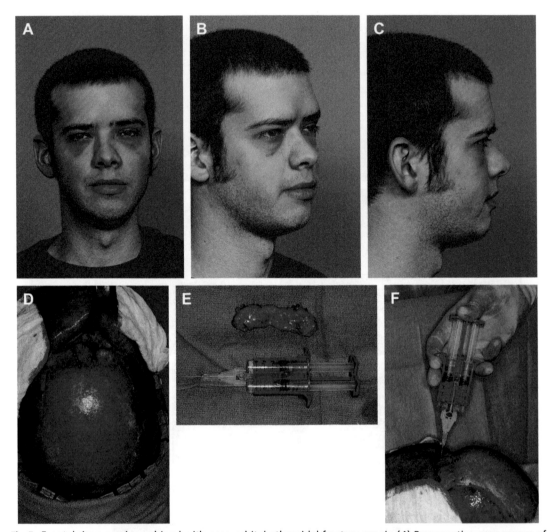

Fig. 5. Frontal sinus repair combined with naso-orbital-ethmoidal fracture repair. (*A*) Preoperative appearance of 19-year-old male following assault with a baseball bat. (*B*) Oblique view showing frontal depression. (*C*) Profile view showing frontonasal depression. (*D*) Surgical exposure via coronal incision. Nasofrontal duct obstruction was noted on exploration. (*E*) Abdominal fat harvest and fibrin glue for obliteration of the frontal sinus. (*F*) Fibrin glue used to seal anterior skull base following removal of all sinus mucosa. (*G*) Pericranial flap harvest. (*H*) Obliteration of frontal sinus with abdominal fat. (*I*) Reduction and stabilization of the anterior table of the frontal sinus using titanium plates and screws. (*J*) Postoperative frontal view. (*K*) Postoperative oblique view. (*L*) Postoperative profile view. Note improved nasal projection.

advantage of being located within the operative field, making harvest convenient, and the available volume is more than adequate. The disadvantage, however, is that the nonvascularized graft undergoes liquefaction necrosis and eventual replacement by fibrous tissue. In addition, donor site morbidity, including temporal hollowing and trismus, are unacceptable, making this technique a poor choice for use in frontal sinus obliteration.

Autogenous bone

Dickenson[55] first described the use of autogenous bone for frontal sinus obliteration in 1969. Since

then, cancellous bone grafts, most often harvested from the ilium, have been widely used as a filler material. Donald and Ettin[58] have shown that when there is loss or comminution of the sinus walls, adipose grafts are less reliable than bone grafts because of loss of adipose graft volume, ingrowth of mucosa, and mucocele formation. Cancellous bone grafts promote reossification from both the periphery of the defect and centrally; therefore, they do not require intact bony walls and will accomplish reossification in a bony cavity. Another advantage of cancellous bone grafts for obliteration is their ability to proliferate and induce

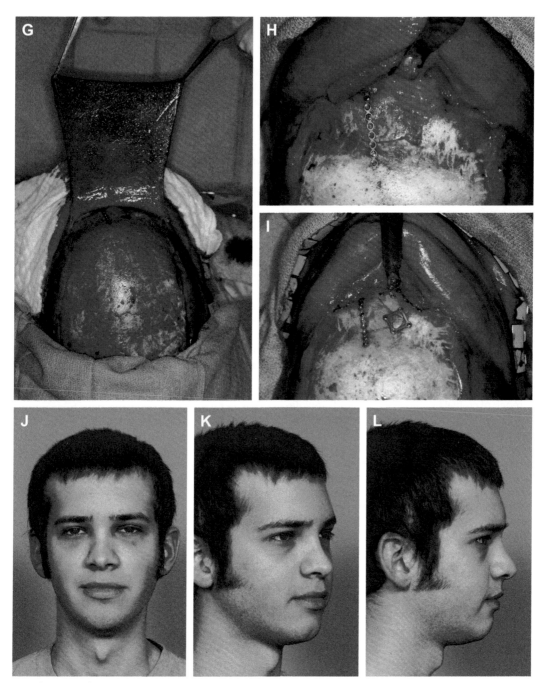

Fig. 5. (*continued*)

bone formation beyond the margins of the original graft and fill the residual dead space through osteogenesis.[59] Another advantage of cancellous bone over adipose tissue for obliteration is that it is easier radiographically to distinguish between resorption, infection, and mucocele formation. The greatest disadvantage to the use of cancellous bone grafts for reconstruction and obliteration lies with the potential donor site morbidity. This can be reduced in the anterior iliac crest bone graft harvest by limiting dissection of the iliacus muscle on the medial aspect of the ilium.

Alloplastic materials

Hydroxyapatite bone cement Commercially available hydroxyapatite cement (BoneSource, Stryker Leibinger, Dallas, Texas) is a nonceramic calcium phosphate preparation that has been advocated by some investigators for use in various craniomaxillofacial surgery applications.[60–62] It has osteoconductive properties, may be contoured to a defect, adheres to adjacent bone, has the ability to resist mucosal ingrowth, is resistant to infection, and is gradually replaced by native bone without a loss of volume. It is currently approved for use by the Food and Drug Administration (FDA) for the repair of cranial burr hole defects and craniofacial skeletal augmentation, and has an excellent record of success in skull molding applications. However, the use of hydroxyapatite cement in the frontal sinus is not recommended. Several investigators have described significant problems related to material failure when this product is in contact with blood, CSF, or other moist conditions, such as those found in the paranasal sinuses.[62–64] Moreover, removal of the degraded material is considerably problematic.

Calcium phosphate bone cement Carbonated calcium phosphate cement (Norion CRS, Norion Corporation, Cupertino, California) differs from hydroxapatite cement in that it is more soluble at low pH, which facilitates resorption and ultimate replacement by bone.[65–68] Although similar in chemical structure to hydroxyapatite, a carbonate substitution of a hydroxyl group makes it more similar to autogenous bone. The cement has osteoconductive characteristics and undergoes a remodeling process similar to that of cortical and cancellous bone. The material is manufactured as a powder that is mixed with sodium phosphate solution to produce an injectable paste that has a working time of approximately 5 minutes before it hardens. Although its handling characteristics make it an ideal alloplastic material, it is particularly prone to degradation and chronic foreign body reactions when placed directly over dura.[69]

Although well suited for cranioplasty applications, its use in the frontal sinus is not recommended (**Fig. 6**).[1]

Glass ionomers Glass ionomer cement is a hybrid glass polymer composite consisting of inorganic glass particles in an insoluble hydrogel matrix and bonded by ionic cross-links, hydrogen bridges, and chain entanglements.[70] It is an osteoconductive material that provides ions for the production of new bone. Glass ionomer cement has a number of advantages over acrylic bone cements. These advantages include the lack of an exothermic reaction, the absence of monomer, and the improved release of incorporated therapeutic agents. Compared with hydroxyapatite, glass ionomer cement results in better bone fill of defects, faster healing time, and faster frontal bone defect occlusion. The histologic fate of the material when placed into the frontal sinus is primarily that of fibroconnective tissue proliferation rather than new bone formation.

Glass ionomer cements are currently the only commercially available alloplast recommended for use in obliteration of the frontal sinus. Several studies have documented favorable results.[71–73] No adverse effects, such as resorption, inflammation, or foreign body reactions, have been reported in clinical or experimental studies. However, one should be careful when interpreting the existing literature. Although favorable short-term results (under 5 years) have been achieved, the long-term fate of these materials when placed in the frontal sinus is not known. Other alloplastic materials have previously held similar promise and subsequently fell into disfavor. Absence of evidence of risk does not mean evidence of absence of risk. Among obliteration materials available for use in the frontal sinus, autogenous

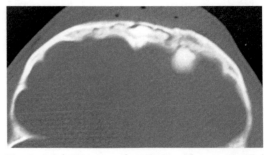

Fig. 6. Axial CT scan of patient with comminuted frontal sinus fractures treated with repair and obliteration with hydroxyapatite cement. Note material failure. The patient required reoperation with debridement of the filler material.

materials, such as abdominal fat, remain the most predictable and the least vulnerable to morbidity.

Cranialization

Frontal sinus cranialization is considered the standard operation for patients with severe head injuries that involve the frontal sinus or anterior skull base (**Figs. 7** and **8**). The procedure is similar to frontal sinus obliteration with the exception that the posterior table is completely removed with a round burr or a Kerrison rongeur. This procedure may be done with the assistance of a neurosurgeon, depending on the extent of underlying brain injury, the presence of dural lacerations, or the need for an extensive craniotomy. It can also be combined with immediate reconstruction of the orbital roof, medial orbit, or naso-orbital-ethmoidal fractures using autogenous bone grafts or alloplastic materials. Once the frontal bone is exposed and the anterior table removed—either by removing the fractured segments or by formal frontal craniotomy—the posterior table is completely removed and the adherent underlying dura or brain is exposed. Care should be taken to maintain the integrity of the cribriform plate, if possible, and to avoid the sagittal sinus where the bone invaginates on either side. Occasionally, it is possible to preserve half of the frontal sinus if the intrasinus septum remains intact and the contralateral sinus remains functionally and anatomically inviolate. Once all the sinus mucosa and the posterior bony table have been removed; the nonviable bone, soft tissue or damaged brain debrided; and dural lacerations repaired, consideration can be given to performing bone graft reconstruction of the orbital roof, naso-orbital-ethmoid complex, or cribriform plate/fovea ethmoidalis, as necessary. A pericranial flap is then rotated into the defect to isolate the splachnocranium from the frontal sinus. The obstructed duct is then sealed with fibrin glue. The brain is allowed to expand into the extradural dead space and the anterior table is reconstructed and stabilized with plates and screws.

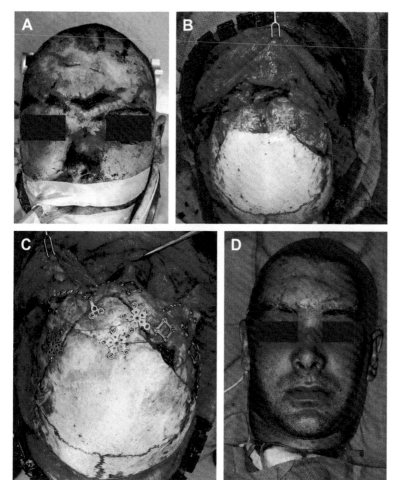

Fig. 7. Cranialization of frontal sinus combined with formal anterior craniotomy and neurosurgical decompression. (*A*) Preoperative appearance of 26-year-old male involved in high-speed motor vehicle collision. (*B*) Intraoperative view of patient following bifrontal craniotomy. The posterior wall of the anterior table is excised, along with all remnants of sinus mucosa. The nasopharynx is separated from the neurocranium by a pericranial flap and fibrin glue. (*C*) The anterior table is replaced and stabilized with titanium plates and screws. (*D*) Postoperative appearance 1 week following surgery.

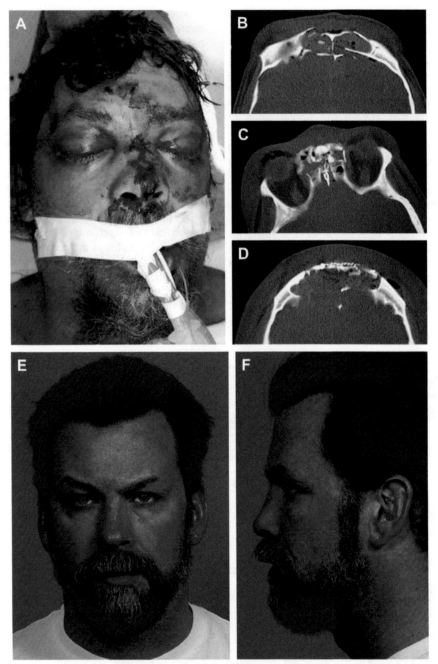

Fig. 8. Cranialization without formal neurosurgical intervention. (*A*) Preoperative appearance of a 42-year-old male following high-speed motor vehicle accident. (*B*) Preoperative axial CT scan showing comminuted anterior and posterior table frontal sinus fractures. (*C*) Preoperative axial CT scan showing complete disruption of the anterior skull base and obstruction of the nasofrontal recess consistent with a Raveh type II injury. (*D*) Axial CT scan obtained 6 months following cranialization of the frontal sinus showing favorable restoration of frontal contour and good bone healing. (*E*) Postoperative frontal view of the patient 12 months after surgery. (*F*) Twelve-month profile view of patient.

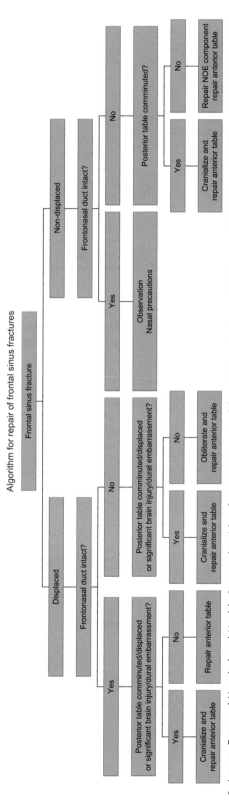

Fig. 9. Legacy Emanuel Hospital and Health Center algorithm for management of frontal sinus fractures. NOE, naso-orbital-ethmoidal. (*From* Bell RB, Dierks EJ, Brar P, et al. A protocol for the management of frontal sinus fractures emphasizing sinus preservation. J Oral Maxillofac Surg 2007;65:825–39; with permission.)

SUMMARY

The previously modified treatment protocols have been developed based on a thorough clinical examination and CT imaging in an attempt to provide a practical and safe rationale for the management of frontal sinus injuries (**Fig. 9**).[74] Once the decision is made to operate, the surgeon must first determine whether to preserve a functional sinus or to separate the sinus from the nasal cavity. Our approach has been to preserve sinus function whenever possible, which is generally indicated for patients with displaced anterior table fractures, no nasofrontal duct involvement, and minimal or no posterior table disruption. Sinus function is maintained by simply repairing the anterior table by stabilizing the bony fragments with low-profile titanium plates and screws or biodegradable fixation. Biodegradable plates and screws are ideal for frontal sinus fractures and provide a safe alternative to the more traditional titanium fixation by virtue of their favorable resorption profiles; adequate strength for use in non-loaded areas, such as the skull; and a long record of success. Although some investigators advocate complete removal of the sinus membrane if it has been violated, we make no effort when preserving the sinus to remove the sinus membrane unless it is diseased or infected.

Patients with displaced anterior tables, evidence of nasofrontal duct obstruction, and little or no posterior table involvement should have the frontal sinus obliterated. Many biomaterials are available for use in frontal sinus obliteration, including autogenous grafts, such as bone, muscle, and fat; and alloplasts, such as methylmethacrylate, hydroxyapatite bone cement (Bone-Source, Stryker Leibinger), calcium phosphate bone cement (Norion, Synthes, Paoli, Pennsylvania), and glass ionomer (Abmin Technologies, Turku, Finland). Obliteration by spontaneous regeneration has also been recommended. While each of these techniques and materials has advocates, autogenous abdominal fat is the most studied material and has the longest record of success. Avoiding donor site morbidity provides much motivation for the use of various alloplastic, bone-substitute materials. However, it is the author's opinion that they should generally be avoided. Neither hydroxyapatite nor calcium phosphate bone cement is approved by the FDA for use in the frontal sinus and there is evidence that complete dissolution of the implant material can occur, leading to mucocele formation eventually requiring implant removal.[65] Studies investigating the use of bioactive glass (glass ionomer cements) have been more favorable, and this material remains the only commercially available bone substitute that is FDA approved for use in the frontal sinus.[71–73] Despite this, we prefer autogenous abdominal fat, which has a long record of safety and, in our experience, has little or no significant donor site morbidity.

Patients who have severely displaced and comminuted frontal sinus fractures with significant posterior table involvement, dural lacerations, persistent CSF leak, or brain injury often benefit from cranialization. Persistent CSF leaks occurring from anterior skull-base fractures are unusual, but may require an intracranial approach that includes dural repair and cranialization of the frontal sinus. CSF leaks in the postoperative setting can most often be treated by bedrest, CSF diversion, and, occasionally, extracranial ethmoid obliteration.[32] From a practical point of view, our own experience and collaboration with neurosurgeons has shown that many patients with significant posterior table displacement require neurosurgical intervention to inspect and repair dura, evacuate hematomas, and debride brain tissue. Formal craniotomy is required in the minority of patients, generally those with rudimentary sinuses, through-and-through or penetrating injuries, or those with massive brain injury. Often the frontal sinus cranialization can be performed via the existing frontal bone fractures or through the posterior sinus wall, and many times the procedure is completed without neurosurgical assistance. A robust pericranial flap should be developed at the time of the coronal approach. This flap is used to line the skull base and plug the nasofrontal recess. Meticulous attention to removal of all sinus mucosa is critical, as is debridement of foreign material or devitalized tissue. If the brain injury is so severe as to warrant a decompressive craniectomy that involves the frontal sinus, the sinus membrane should be removed, a peripheral ostectomy performed, and the frontal bone reconstructed at a later date.

REFERENCES

1. Stanley RB. Fractures of the frontal sinus. Clin Plast Surg 1989;16(1):115.
2. Reidel. In Schenke: inaug dissertation. Jena, 1898.
3. Killian G. Die Killianische Radicaloperation chronischer stirnhohleneiterungen: II. Weiteres kasuistisches material und zusammenfassung. Arch Laryngo Rhinol 1904;13:59 [German].
4. Lynch RC. The technique of a radical frontal sinus operation which has given me the best results. Laryngoscope 1921;31:1–5.
5. Bergara A, Itioz O. Experimental study of the behavior of adipose tissue within the frontal sinus

of the dog. Argent Rev Oto Rhinolaryngol 1951;184: 184–92.

6. Bergara AR, Itoiz OA. Present state of the surgical treatment of chronic frontal sinusitis. Arch Otolaryngol 1955;61:616–28.

7. Montgomery WW. The fate of adipose implants in a bony cavity. Laryngoscope 1964;74:816–27.

8. Goodale RL, Montgomery WW. Experiences with the osteoplastic anterior wall approach to the frontal sinus; case histories and recommendations. Arch Otolaryngol 1958;68:271–83.

9. Nadell J, Kline DG. Primary reconstruction on depressed frontal sinus fractures including those involving the sinus, orbit and cribriform plate. J Neurosurg 1974;41:200–7.

10. Donald PJ, Bernstein L. Compound frontal sinus injuries with intracranial penetration. Laryngoscope 1978;88(2):225–32.

11. Donald PJ. Frontal sinus ablation by cranialization: a report of 21 cases. Arch Otolaryngol 1982;108:142–6.

12. Whited RE. Anterior table frontal sinus fractures. Laryngoscope 1979;89:1951–5.

13. Larrabee WF, Travis LW, Tabb HG. Frontal sinus fractures: their suppurative complications and surgical management. Laryngoscope 1980;90:1810–3.

14. Sataloff RT, Sariego J, Meyers DL, et al. Surgical management of the frontal sinus. Neurosurgery 1984;15:593.

15. Stanley RB, Becker TS. Injuries of the nasofrontal orifices in frontal sinus fractures. Laryngoscope 1987;97:728–31.

16. Luce EA. Frontal sinus fractures: guidelines to management. Plast Reconstr Surg 1987;80:500–8.

17. Wolfe SA, Johnson P. Frontal sinus injuries: primary care and management of late complications. Plast Reconstr Surg 1988;82:781–9.

18. Wallis A, Donald PJ. Frontal sinus fractures: a review of 72 cases. Laryngoscope 1988;98:593–8.

19. Rohrich RJ, Hollier LH. Management of frontal sinus fractures: changing concepts. Clin Plast Surg 1992; 19:219–32.

20. Helmy ES, Koh ML, Bays RA. Management of frontal sinus fractures: review of the literature and clinical update. Oral Surg Oral Med Oral Pathol 1990;69: 137–48.

21. Klotch DW. Frontal sinus fractures: anterior skull base. Facial Plast Surg 2000;16(2):127–33.

22. Kalavrezos N. Current trends in the management of frontal sinus fractures. Injury 2004;35:340–6.

23. Rice DH. Management of frontal sinus fractures. Curr Opin Otolaryngol Head Neck Surg 2004;12:46–8.

24. Swinson BD, Jerjes W, Thompson G. Current practice in the management of frontal sinus fractures. J Laryngol Otol 2004;118:927–32.

25. Haug RH, Cunningham LL. Management of fractures of the frontal bone and frontal sinus. Selected Readings Oral Maxillofac Surg. Vol. 10, No 6 2002.

26. Tiwari P, Higuera S, Thornton J, et al. The management of frontal sinus fractures. J Oral Maxillofac Surg 2005;63(9):1354–60.

27. Tato JM, Sibbald DW, Bergaglio OE. Surgical treatment of the frontal sinus by the external route. Laryngoscope 1954;64:504–21.

28. McHugh HE. Treatment of the fractures of the frontal and ethmoid sinuses. Laryngoscope 1958;68:1616–40.

29. Newman MH, Travis LW. Frontal sinus fractures. Laryngoscope 1973;83:1281–92.

30. Hybels RL, Newman MH. Posterior table fractures of the frontal sinus: II. Clinical aspects. Laryngoscope 1977;87:1740–5.

31. Gonty AA, Marciani RD, Adornato DC. Management of frontal sinus fractures: a review of 33 cases. J Oral Maxillofac Surg 1999;57:372–9.

32. Bell RB, Dierks EJ, Homer L, et al. Management of cerebrospinal fluid leaks associated with craniomaxillofacial trauma. J Oral Maxillofac Surg 2004;62: 676–84, 21.

33. Manolidis S. Frontal sinus injuries: associated injuries and surgical management of 93 patients. J Oral Maxillofac Surg 2004;62:882–91.

34. Xie C, Mehendale N, Barrett D, et al. 30-year retrospective review of frontal sinus fractures: the Charity Hospital experience. J Craniomaxillofac Trauma 2000;6(1):7–15.

35. Heller EM, Jacobs JB, Holliday RA. Evaluation of the frontonasal duct in frontal sinus fractures. Head Neck 1989;11:46–50.

36. Day TA, Meehan R, Stucker FJ, et al. Management of frontal sinus fractures with posterior table involvement: a retrospective study. J Craniomaxillofac Trauma 1998;4(3):6–9.

37. El Khatib K, Danino A, Malka G. The frontal sinus: a culprit or a victim? A review of 40 cases. J Craniomaxillofac Surg 2004;32:314–7.

38. Gerbino G, Roccia F, Benech A, et al. Analysis of 158 frontal sinus fractures: current surgical management and complications. J Craniomaxillofac Surg 2000;28:133–9.

39. Wright DL, Hoffman HT, Hoyt DB. Frontal sinus fractures in the pediatric population. Laryngoscope 1992;102:1215–9.

40. Ioannides C, Freihofer HP, Friens J. Fractures of the frontal sinus: a rationale of treatment. Br J Plast Surg 1993;46:208–14.

41. Raveh J, Laedrach K, Vuillemin R, et al. Management of combined frontonaso-orbital/skull base fractures and telecanthus in 355 cases. Arch Otolaryngol Head Neck Surg 1992;118:605–14.

42. Bell RB, Kindsfater C. The use of biodegradable plates and screws to stabilize facial fractures. J Oral Maxillofac Surg 2006;64:31–9.

43. Graham HD 3rd, Spring P. Endoscopic repair of frontal sinus fracture: case report. J Craniomaxillofac Trauma 1996;2(4):52–5.

44. Lappert PW, Lee JW. Treatment of an isolated outer table frontal sinus fracture using endoscopic reduction and fixation. Plast Reconstr Surg 1998;102(5):1642–5.

45. Shumrick KA, Ryzenman JM. Endoscopic management of facial fractures. Facial Plast Surg Clin North Am 2001;9(3):469–74.

46. Strong EB, Buchalter GM, Moulthrop TH. Endoscopic repair of isolated anterior table frontal sinus fractures. Arch Facial Plast Surg 2003;5(6):514–21.

47. Chen DJ, Chen CT, Chen YR, et al. Endoscopically assisted repair of frontal sinus fractures. J Trauma 2003;55(2):378–82.

48. Schon R, Gellrich NC, Schmelzeisen R. Frontiers in maxillofacial endoscopic surgery. Atlas Oral Maxillofac Surg Clin North Am 2003;11(2):209–39.

49. Strong EB, Kellman RM. Endoscopic repair of anterior table-frontal sinus fractures. Facial Plast Surg Clin North Am 2006;14(1):25–9.

50. Shumrick KA. Endoscopic management of frontal sinus fractures. Otolaryngol Clin North Am 2007;40(2):329–36.

51. Kim KK, Mueller R, Huang F, et al. Endoscopic repair of anterior table: frontal sinus fractures with a Medpor implant. Otolaryngol Head Neck Surg 2007;136(4):568–72.

52. Yoo MH, Kim JS, Song HM, et al. Endoscopic transnasal reduction of an anterior table frontal sinus fracture: technical note. Int J Oral Maxillofac Surg 2008;37(6):573–5.

53. D'Addario M, Haug RH, Talwar RM. Biomaterials for use in frontal sinus obliteration. J Long Term Eff Med Implants 2004;14(6):455–65.

54. Wilson BC, Davidson B, Corey JP, et al. Comparison of complications following frontal sinus fractures managede with exploration with or without obliteration over 10 years. Laryngoscope 1988;98:516–20.

55. Dickenson JT, Capic JA, Kameron DB. Principles of frontal reconstruction. Laryngoscope 1969;79(6):1019–75.

56. Mickel TJ, Rohrich RJ, Robinson JB. Frontal sinus obliteration: a comparison of fat, bone, muscle and spontaneous osteogenesis in the cat model. Plast Reconstr Surg 1990;5(3):586–92.

57. Rohrich RJ, Mickel TJ. Frontal sinus obliteration: in search of the ideal material. Plast Reconstr Surg 1995;95(3):580–5.

58. Donald PJ, Ettin M. The safety of frontal sinus fat obliteraion when sinus walls are missing. Laryngoscope 1986;96:190–3.

59. Shumrick KA, Smith CP. The use of cancellous bone for frontal sinus obliteration and reconstruction of frontal bony defects. Arch Otolaryngol Head Neck Surg 1994;120:1003–9.

60. Kent JN, Zide MF, Kay JF, et al. Hydroxyapatite blocks and particles as bone graft substitutes in orthognathic and reconstructive surgery. J Oral Maxillofac Surg 1986;44(8):597–605.

61. Friedman CD, Costantino PD, Jones K, et al. Hydroxyapatite cement II: obliteration and reconstruction of the cat frontal sinus. Arch Otolaryngol Head Neck Surg 1991;117(4):385–9.

62. Freidman CD, Costantino PD, Snyderman CH, et al. Reconstruction of the frontal sinus and frontofacial skeleton with hydroxyapatite cement. Arch Facial Plast Surg 2000;2(2):124–9.

63. Maniker A, Cantrell S, Vaicys C. Failure of hydroxyapatite cement to set in repair of a cranial defect: case report. Neurosurgery 1998;43(4):953–5.

64. Kveton JF, Friedman CD, Piepmeier JM, et al. Reconstruction of suboccipital craniectomy defects with hydroxyapatite cement: a preliminary report. Laryngoscope 1995;105(2):156–9.

65. Verret DJ, Ducic Y, Oxford L, et al. Hydroxyapatite cement in craniofacial reconstruction. Otolaryngol Head Neck Surg 2005;133(6):897–9.

66. Frankenburg EP, Goldstein SA, Bauer TW, et al. Biomechanical and histological evaluation of a calcium phosphate cement. J Bone Joint Surg Am 1998;80(8):1112–24.

67. Baker SB, Weinzweig J, Kirschner RE, et al. Applications of a new carbonated calcium phosphate bone cement: early experience in pediatric and adult craniofacial reconstruction. Plast Reconstr Surg 2002;109(6):1789–90.

68. Mahr MA, Bartley GB, Bite U, et al. Norion craniofacial repair bone cement for the repair of craniofacial skeletal defects. Ophthal Plast Reconstr Surg 2000;16(5):393–8.

69. Matic D, Phillips JH. A contraindication for the use of hydroxyapatite cement in the pediatric population. Plast Reconstr Surg 2002;110(1):1–5.

70. McClean JW. Glass-ionomer cements. Braz Dent J 1988;164:292–300.

71. Peltola MJ, Suonpaa JT, Aitasalo KMJ, et al. Experimental follow-up model for clinical frontal sinus obliteration with bioactive glass (S53P4). Acta Otolaryngol Suppl 2000;54:167–9.

72. Peltola MJ, Suonpaa JT, Maattanen HS, et al. Clinical follow-up method for frontal sinus obliteration with bioactive glass S53P4. J Biomed Mater Res 2001;58(1):54–60.

73. Peltola M, Suonpaa J, Aitasalo K, et al. Obliteration of the frontal sinus cavity with bioactive glass. Head Neck 1998;20(4):315–9.

74. Bell RB, Dierks EJ, Brar P, et al. A protocol for the management of frontal sinus fractures emphasizing sinus preservation. J Oral Maxillofac Surg 2007;65:825–39.

Management of Parotid Gland and Duct Injuries

Joseph E. Van Sickels, DDS

KEYWORDS

• Management • Injury • Parotid duct • Parotid gland

Surgical repair of injuries to the parotid gland and its duct have been described in the literature for more than 100 years.[1] Injury to the glandular structures are usually associated with penetrating wounds of the face and often involve concomitant damage to adjacent structures, including the facial nerve, the ear, and the nearby bony structures (**Fig. 1**).[2,3] Most investigators agree that management of these injuries depends on the location of the damage. However, there are differences of opinion as to the proper management of the repair when the injury to the glandular system is discovered early or late.[1–6]

DIAGNOSIS

Any penetrating injury along a line drawn from the tragus of the ear to the midportion of the upper lip may injure either Stenson's duct or the parotid gland.[1] Van Sickels and Alexander,[6] and later Stevenson,[7] noted that the glandular system can be injured in three different regions. Region A is the area of the gland (**Fig. 2**), region B is the site of the duct as it runs superficial to the masseter muscle, and region C is the region from the masseter muscle to where it enters the oral cavity in the buccal mucosa opposite the maxillary second molar.[7]

The buccal branch of the facial nerve often runs with the duct, which crosses the superficial layer of the masseter after it exits the parotid gland (**Fig. 3**). When the nerve is injured, the patient may present with weakness of the upper lip when trying to animate. Intraoperatively, the wound should be explored and the duct cannulated. Although some investigators suggest that a toluidine blue dye should be injected into the duct to help identify the proximal end, the author feels that a transection of the duct can be seen without the injection of a dye.[3] Especially with a dark-colored dye, excessive extravasation from the lacerated duct may complicate surgery because of discoloration of the surgical field. Rather than a dye, saline can be injected if difficulty is encountered in finding the proximal end. No fluid seen in the wound indicates that the duct is intact.

Timing of Repair

Most investigators believe that the repair should be done early, preferably in the first 24 hours.[2,6] This is because late complications, such as a parotid fistula, are difficult to treat (see section below). Cannulation of the duct also becomes more difficult as the swelling increases, making determination of the status of the duct a more complex task.

However, some investigators do not feel that immediate repair of the duct is always necessary. Lewis and Knottenbelt[8] treated 33 patients seen in a 6-month period who had parotid gland or duct injury, most caused by sharp injury or a low velocity gun shot. All had wound closure without direct repair of the duct, and all but three had follow-up sialograms. There were no clinical complications in nine of the 19 patients who had follow-up. Complications seen in the remaining 10 were salivary fistula (seven patients) and sialoceles (four patients), but all eventually healed without surgical management. Although healing occurred, it involved a prolonged course, and it is likely that most of these complications could have been avoided by early treatment.

Division of Oral and Maxillofacial Surgery, University of Kentucky, Lexington, KY 40536-0297, USA
E-mail address: vansick@email.uky.edu

Oral Maxillofacial Surg Clin N Am 21 (2009) 243–246
doi:10.1016/j.coms.2008.12.010

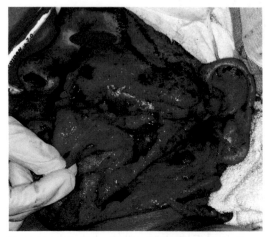

Fig. 1. Complex laceration of overlying soft tissue, parotid duct and gland (regions A and B) with an auricle laceration and fracture of mandible.

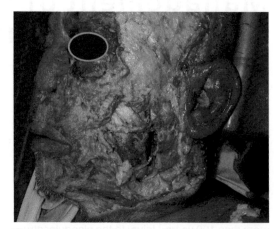

Fig. 3. Anatomic dissection illustrating the duct running over the masseter approximately along a line drawn from the tragus of the ear to the midportion of the upper lip.

MANAGEMENT OF INJURIES TO THE GLAND AND DUCT

Injury to the gland alone generally involves repair of the injury, putting a stent in the duct, and placing a pressure dressing.[2,3] The stent keeps the duct patent during the time the pressure dressing is in place. The main surgical options for injury to the duct include repair of the duct over a stent, ligation of the duct, or fistulization of the duct into the oral cavity.[4–6] When a stent is inserted, most investigators leave it in place for a period of weeks;[4,6] however, Stevenson[7] and Sparkman[9] suggest that it is not necessary to leave the stent in place once the parotid duct is repaired.

When there are extensive injuries to the glandular/duct system and both ends of the duct cannot be found or are macerated, ligation of the proximal portion of the duct is recommended, the

theory being that the gland will undergo atrophy.[4,6] Findings of one animal study have suggested that an injury to the duct with a resultant continuity defect can be repaired with an autogenous graft.[10] In contrast, others have shown that continuity defects repaired with an autogenous graft generally are unsuccessful.[11] Injury of the orifice of the duct where it enters the oral cavity often is managed by insertion of a drain (Fig. 4A, B). The concept is that saliva will drain into the oral cavity, and a new orifice will be created.

COMPLICATIONS

Injuries to the parotid glandular system can be missed as the result of extensive trauma, subsequently resulting in sialoceles, parotid fistulae, and infections.[3,8,12] They may also occur when repair of an injury is not successful. Medical management of such conditions includes antisialogogues and antibiotics.[3] Antisialogogues often are combined with aspiration from a nondependent area and application of a pressure dressing when there is a fluid collection or a sialocele occurs. Botulinum toxin has been used for salivary fistulas caused by a number of different problems.[12–14] Breuer and colleagues[12] reported two cases of salivary fistula after facial trauma, one of which was from the parotid. In both instances they were successful in treating the fistula with the injection of botulinum toxin into the gland. Some investigators have reported good results treating delayed fistulas and sialoceles by other means.[15–18] One course of therapy consisted of restricting all oral intake, giving an antisialogogue, placing a pressure dressing, and keeping the patient on intravenous fluids for 5 days.[15] In these

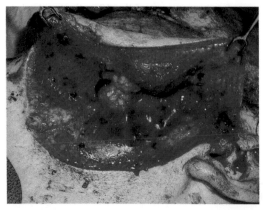

Fig. 2. Penetrating laceration of face over the region of the duct.

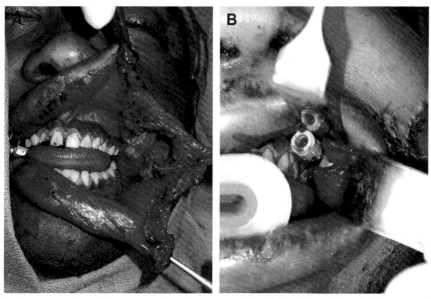

Fig. 4. (*A*) Gunshot wound entering near orifice of Stenson's duct. (*B*) Drain in place, left for 2 weeks.

different studies it was noted that injuries over the gland region (region A) responded more quickly than those that occurred over the region of the duct (region B). Another approach is to do a tympanic neurectomy or parotidectomy for chronic parotid gland problems; this therapy can also be used for chronic fistulae.[17,18]

SUMMARY

Unfortunately, most of the information on the management of parotid gland and duct injuries is based on relatively small clinical studies. However, the preponderance of these studies suggests that the injuries in this region should be treated early and that that the location of the injury has bearing on the type of treatment. Injuries to the glandular portion (region A) should be treated by meticulous closure and a pressure dressing with or without stenting Stenson's duct. Treatment of the duct region is slightly controversial, with most investigators suggesting that the wound should be closed with a stent in the duct, even if it is intact, because subsequent swelling can still cause obstruction. In contrast, Lewis and Knottenbelt suggest that this is not necessary.[8] However, when examining their data, three of those with a region B injury had a sialocele, and four had a salivary fistula (one patient had both). Only two patients with a region B injury had an uncomplicated course. Although they were able to successfully manage all of their complications, their data suggest that it may be better to recognize and treat the problem when the patient initially presents for therapy. Injury to the orifice of the duct is usually treated by placing a drain.

When chronic conditions arise, such as sialoceles or fistulas, management becomes more complicated. Traditional therapy for sialoceles includes aspiration from a nondependent aspect accompanied by a pressure dressing. In the author's experience, this may require multiple aspirations, with or without use of adjunctive medications. Fistulas are more challenging to treat. Although multiple surgical and medical therapies have been proposed to treat them, resolving a chronic fistula is sometimes difficult. Use of botulinum toxin injection into the glandular structure alone or with other therapies appears to be very promising.

REFERENCES

1. Revis DR, Seagle MB. Parotid duct injures. eMedicine August 1, 2006; last update.
2. Tachmes L, Woloszyn T, Marini C, et al. Parotid gland and facial nerve trauma: a retrospective review. J Trauma 1990;30:1395–8.
3. Lewkowicz AA, Hasson O, Nablieli O. Traumatic injuries to the parotid gland and duct. J Oral Maxillofac Surg 2002;60:676–80.
4. Epker BN, Burnette JC. Trauma to the parotid gland and duct: primary treatment and management of complications. J Oral Surg 1970;28:657–70.
5. Steinberg MJ, Herrera AF. Management of parotid duct injuries. Oral Surg Oral Med Oral Pathol Oral Radiol Endod 2005;99:136–41.
6. Van Sickels JE, Alexander JM. Parotid duct injuries. Oral Surg 1981;52:364–7.

7. Stevenson JH. Parotid duct transection associated with facial trauma: experience with 10 cases. Br J Plast Surg 1983;36:81–3.

8. Lewis G, Knottenbelt JD. Parotid duct injury: is immediate surgical repair necessary? Injury 1991; 22:407–9.

9. Sparkman RS. Laceration of parotid duct further experiences. Ann Surg 1950;131:743–54.

10. Chudakov O, Ludchik T. Microsurgical repair of Stensen's and Wharton's ducts with autogenous venous grafts. An experimental study on dogs. Int J Oral Maxillofac Surg 1999;28:70–3.

11. Dumpis J, Feldmane L. Experimental microsurgery of salivary ducts in dogs. J Craniomaxillofac Surg 2001;29:56–62.

12. Breuer T, Ferrazzini A, Grossenbacher R. Botulinum toxin A as a treatment of traumatic salivary gland fistulas. HNO 2006;54:385–90.

13. Marchese-Ragona R, Marioni G, Restivo DA, et al. The role of botulium toxin in post parotidectomy fistula treatment. A technical note. Am J Otol 2006; 27:221–4.

14. Lim YC, Choi EC. Treatment of an acute salivary fistula after parotid surgery: botulinum toxin type A injection as primary treatment. Eur Arch Otorhinolaryngol 2008;265:243–5.

15. Landau R, Stewart M. Conservative management of post-traumatic parotid fistulae and sialoceles: a prospective study. Br J Surg 1985; 72:42–4.

16. Parekh D, Glezerson G, Stewart M, et al. Post-traumatic parotid fistulae and sialoceles. A prospective study of conservative management in 51 cases. Ann Surg 1989;209:105–11.

17. Perera AM, Kumar BN, Pahor AL. Long-term results of tympanic neurectomy for chronic parotid sialectasis. Rev Laryngol Otol Rhinol (Bord) 2000;121: 95–8.

18. Vasama JP. Tympanic neurectomy and chronic parotitis. Acta Otolaryngol 2000;120:995–8.

Management of Facial Bite Wounds

Panagiotis K. Stefanopoulos, DDS, MAJ (DC)*

KEYWORDS

- Bite wound • Facial injury • Animal bite
- Human bite • Soft-tissue infection

Bite wounds have always been considered complex injuries contaminated with a unique polymicrobial inoculum. Because wounds of the extremities constitute the majority of bite cases, most relevant studies have focused on the wound infection rate in these areas. However, a substantial subset of dog, cat, and human bites, each in the order of 15%, are located on the face,[1–4] where fear of potential disfigurement is an overriding concern and the associated psychological consequences can be devastating.[5]

Although a wide range of mammals have been implicated in facial bite injuries,[6–13] the majority of these injuries are inflicted by dogs.[6,9,12,13] It is estimated that there are 44,000 facial injuries from dog bites affecting children each year in the United States.[3–5,9,12,14–22] Not surprisingly, facial injuries predominate in those dog-bite casualties requiring hospitalization.[14,20]

For half a century, oral and maxillofacial surgeons have remained in the forefront of the surgical treatment of these injuries.[12,23–27] Nevertheless, certain aspects of therapy remain amenable to personal opinions and clinical impressions.[18,28] The aim of this article is to discuss these issues in the general context of bite-wound management (**Box 1**), including the role of prophylactic antibiotics and the possible limitations of the general axiom of primary closure.

WOUND CHARACTERISTICS

Animal bites can result in three main types of soft tissue trauma, namely punctures, lacerations, and avulsions, with or without an actual tissue defect.[14,23,29–31] The typical dog bite results in a combination of torn tissues and adjacent punctures, the so-called "hole-and-tear" effect (**Fig. 1**).[32] Some degree of crush injury is also present in most bite wounds, including those from humans, due to the dynamics of the bite.[27,33] Dog bites of the face are located mostly on the lips, nose, or cheeks.[12,14,15,18,21,34–36] Human bites notably tend to involve the ear,[24,31,37,38] although the lower lip is also prominently involved.[24,39–43]

Bite wounds inflicted to the head and neck region by large animals can present in a more serious fashion.[7,10,11] Large dog attacks can result in life-threatening or even fatal injuries because of airway compromise, exsanguination, or craniocerebral trauma.[22,44–46] Furthermore, dog bites can impart enough energy to the facial skeleton to cause structural damage, especially in children.[15,29,46,47]

OVERVIEW OF MICROBIOLOGY

The importance of the indigenous oral bacteria in bite-wound infections is substantiated by the high isolation rates (>50% of cases) of *Pasteurella* spp from dog and cat bites,[33,48,49] and viridans streptococci, especially *Streptococcus anginosus*, from human bites.[30] There are also corresponding figures for oral anaerobes, including *Fusobacterium nucleatum*, *Bacteroides*, *Prevotella*, and *Porphyromonas* spp.[12,30,49] It should be appreciated, however, that almost any oral organism can become a potential pathogen under the right circumstances.[50]

Consistent with the heterogeneity observed between feline and canine oropharyngeal *Pasteurella* strains,[51] *P canis* biotype 1 is the predominant isolate from dog bites, whereas *P multocida* subspecies *multocida* and *septica* have been

Dental Corps, Hellenic Army, Oral and Maxillofacial Surgery Department, 401 Army Hospital, Mesogeion & Katehaki Ave, Athens 11525, Greece
* Corresponding author. 88 Pontou Street, Goudi, Athens 11527, Greece.
E-mail address: pstefanopoulos@yahoo.com

Oral Maxillofacial Surg Clin N Am 21 (2009) 247–257
doi:10.1016/j.coms.2008.12.009
1042-3699/08/$ – see front matter © 2009 Elsevier Inc. All rights reserved.

Box 1
Controversial topics in the management of facial bite wounds

- Selection of solution for wound irrigation
- Irrigation of puncture wounds
- Role of antibiotic prophylaxis
- Selection of antimicrobial agent(s)
- Cutoff time for primary closure

isolated much more frequently from cat bites.[49,52] Streptococci and staphylococci are the next most common aerobic isolates.[49,53] Potentially invasive aerobic organisms isolated from domestic animal bites include *Bergeyella* (*Weeksella*) *zoohelcum* and *Capnocytophaga canimorsus*, the latter associated with fulminant systemic infections in immunocompromised hosts, usually after a dog bite.[49,54–56]

Staphylococci are also commonly isolated from human bites.[30,53,57] *Eikenella corrodens*, a normal inhabitant of the human oral cavity, appears to have a unique association with human bites, having been recovered from about 30% of cases.[30] Other fastidious gram-negative organisms, such as *Haemophilus* spp and enteric gram-negative rods, have been found less frequently.[30,57] Oral as well as environmental fungi may also contaminate bite wounds.[54] *Candida* spp have been isolated from 8% of infected human bites, but their pathogenic role remains unclear.[30]

Bites can also impart systemic bacterial and viral infections, including classic zoonoses.[58] Human bites can be the source of the hepatitis B and C virus, and possibly HIV transmission, as well as syphilis.[27,59] Rabies remains the most dreaded of all animal bite-wound infections, which should be especially considered when bites from bats, raccoons, or foxes are encountered.[27,59,60]

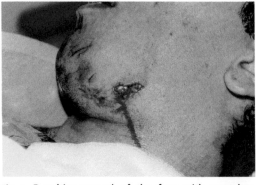

Fig. 1. Dog-bite wound of the face with scratches, punctures, and laceration ("hole-and-tear" effect).

RISK FACTORS FOR WOUND INFECTION

Facial bite wounds generally display low infection rates, commonly attributed to the rich blood supply of the area.[2,18,55,61] Dog bites on the face are usually considered to be at moderate risk for infection when compared with other types of mammalian bites,[33] especially those inflicted by cats,[6,12] which harbor the more toxic *P multocida* organisms.[52] Furthermore, dog-bite wounds seen within 3 hours of injury rarely contain more than 10^5 bacteria per gram of tissue, while human bites usually exceed this critical level[62] because of higher bacterial counts in saliva.[63]

Significant delays–beyond 6 to 12 hours–in seeking medical attention increase the likelihood of infection.[12,22,31,38,39,64–66] Victims of bites to the face are more likely to present in time for prompt wound care than do other bite victims, because of concern about possible scarring.[16,21] However, long delays may be encountered with facial bites, due to alcohol intoxication of the victim[31] or transport from remote areas.[42] Furthermore, prolonged exposure of the wound to bacterial contamination can affect the therapeutic efficacy of antibiotics.[64,67] Unfortunately, no study has controlled for the time from wounding to antibiotic treatment.[68]

Puncture wounds, typically inflicted by the slender feline teeth, are associated with high infection rates because they involve deep inoculation of pathogens.[12,44,69,70] Crush injuries, on the other hand, can precipitate infection with significantly lower bacterial counts because of the resultant tissue ischemia.[57,64,69,71] However, due to the inevitable cartilage exposure, avulsion injuries of the ear or nose inflicted by humans have the highest incidence of infection following facial bite wounds, according to reports.[38]

CLINICAL EVALUATION

With extensive head or neck injury, life-preserving emergency procedures take precedence;[11,22,27,28,46,59,70,72] cervical immobilization should also be considered.[22] Otherwise, there is time to obtain the necessary information about the incident as well as about the general condition of the patient.[44,70]

When there is a possibility of involvement of underlying specialized structures, early diagnosis is essential. Eyelid lacerations require careful evaluation to rule out penetrating injury to the globe or interruption of the lacrimal drainage system.[59,73,74] Radiographic examination of the adjacent facial or cranial bones is indicated when a fracture is suspected.[15,22,75,76] A proposed classification of facial bite wounds,[15,77] based on extent, appears in **Table 1**.

The wound should be assessed for signs of infection, including redness, swelling, or discharge. These signs tend to be more obvious with older wounds than with fresh ones.[12,49] Fever is generally unlikely.[44,48,78,79] P multocida organisms are associated with a rapid onset of infection,[52,78] whereas when the latency period is more than 24 hours, staphylococci, streptococci, or anaerobes are more likely etiologic agents.[22,49,72,79] Cultures are most useful in case initial antibiotic therapy fails.[69]

Bite wounds are considered tetanus-prone,[11,59,72] so appropriate immunization should be administered if the patient has had fewer than three doses of tetanus toxoid or more than 5 years have passed since the last dose.[80–82] Rabies prophylaxis should be based on the local prevalence of the disease, the biting species, and the circumstances surrounding the incident.[44,50,58,59,79,82]

Superficial bite wounds can be treated in the outpatient setting, whereas patients with more serious injuries (types III and IV) should be hospitalized and treated in the operating room. For children whose wounds require surgical care, hospitalization should be considered because they may be uncooperative under local anesthesia.[15,77] Signs of systemic toxicity, rapidly advancing cellulitis, or infection despite oral antibiotic therapy constitute other indications for hospitalization.[56,76] Most adults with uncomplicated bite wounds (type II) can be discharged after wound repair with instructions for follow-up.[77]

LOCAL WOUND CARE

As with any laceration, the mainstays of wound care are irrigation and removal of any necrotic tissue.[58,72,75] However, common practices, such as cleansing with soap or scrubbing,[44,58] are best reserved for high-risk wounds. Irrigation is essential in preventing infection because it removes debris and microorganisms;[59,61,71,72,75,83,84] wounds difficult to irrigate thoroughly, such as punctures, are twice as likely to become infected.[85] Manual irrigation with a 19-gauge catheter on a 30- to 60-mL syringe delivers a pressure range between 5 and 8 psi, considered optimal for appropriate decontamination.[83,84,86,87] Continuous irrigation seems to be just as effective as pulsatile lavage.[86] However, sustained high-pressure irrigation should be avoided in areas containing loose areolar tissue, such as the eyelids or children's cheeks, because such irrigation may cause tissue disruption and excessive edema.[72] In general, 250 to 500 mL of solution provides an adequate cleansing effect for most facial bite wounds.[75,88] Although irrigation of puncture wounds remains controversial because of the inherent difficulties in proper drainage,[72] most investigators also use pressure irrigation for these wounds, taking care to allow escape of the fluid (**Box 2**).[12,44,88] Incising the puncture to promote irrigation[27] is not recommended, however, as it causes unnecessary scarring.[16]

Normal saline is the fluid of choice for irrigation, according to many experts.[16,22,44,72,75,76,84,86,88] A 1% povidone-iodine solution also has been recommended for irrigation of bite wounds because this solution provides an optimal therapeutic balance between bactericidal capacity and tissue toxicity associated with iodine-containing

Table 1	
Classification of facial bite injuries	
Type	**Clinical Findings**
I	Superficial injury without muscle involvement
IIA	Deep injury with muscle involvement
IIB	Full-thickness injury of the cheek or lip with oral mucosal involvement (through-and-through wound)
IIIA	Deep injury with tissue defect (complete avulsion)
IIIB	Deep avulsive injury exposing nasal or auricular cartilage
IVA	Deep injury with severed facial nerve and/or parotid duct
IVB	Deep injury with concomitant bone fracture

From Stefanopoulos PK, Tarantzopoulou AD. Facial bite wounds: management update. Int J Oral Maxillofac Surg 2005;34:469. (*Modified from* Lackmann GM, Draf W, Isselstein G, et al. Surgical treatment of facial dog bite injuries in children. J Craniomaxillofac Surg 1992;20:85; with permission.)

Box 2
Treatment protocol for common facial bite wounds

1. Skin preparation; anesthesia
2. Pressure irrigation; irrigation of puncture wounds
3. Resection of skin tags
4. Removal of visible foreign particles
5. Suturing (exceptions listed below)
6. Consideration of tetanus prophylaxis
7. Follow-up within 24 to 48 hours

Also recommended:

Normal saline irrigation (1% povidone-iodine should be reserved for grossly contaminated wounds)

Antibiotic prophylaxis

Culture of problematic wounds (failure to respond to initial antibiotic therapy or presence of serious infection)

Not recommended:

Routine debridement (if attempted, it should not exceed 1 mm of tissue)

Suturing in the presence of overt infection, gross edema, foreign bodies, or visible contamination (consider delayed closure)

Culture of fresh uninfected wounds, because it depicts the polymicrobial flora of the wound rather than the causative organisms of any subsequent infection

---

formulations.[33,69,79,87] However, when used under pressure for wound decontamination, saline has compared favorably with 1% povidone-iodine solution and other less commonly used alternatives.[89,90] Moreover, even if povidone-iodine or another antiseptic solution is used as an irrigant, copious rinsing with normal saline should follow to minimize the risk of cytotoxicity.[12,15,27]

Surgical debridement is a common clinical practice in bite-wound management[16,37,40,88] because it significantly decreases the likelihood of infection.[57,85] However, debridement of facial wounds should be kept to a minimum so as to avoid sacrifice of tissue that has a good chance to survive,[12,34,38,56] particularly in landmark areas such as the vermilion border of the lips, the nasolabial fold, and the eyebrows (**Box 2**).[25,42,59,75]

SURGICAL TREATMENT

Primary wound closure is the treatment of choice for all uninfected facial bite lacerations seen within 24 hours, as well as for many avulsion injuries, because this obtains the most favorable esthetic result.[12,16–18,26–28,34–36,39–43,59,64,75,91]

Subcutaneous sutures should be used sparingly, however, because they can act as foreign bodies and precipitate infection.[27,59] By contrast, deep puncture wounds should be left open, particularly when inflicted by cats.[27,59]

In the study of Maimaris and Quinton,[65] 1 of 27 sutured wounds in the face became infected compared with none of the 14 wounds left open, a difference considered both insignificant and acceptable in view of the better cosmetic result achieved with suturing. Several other studies have confirmed the low risk associated with suturing of facial bite wounds,[2,41,88,92] although in some studies increased infection rates were found both with dog bites[12,46] and human bites.[38]

For uncomplicated bite wounds presenting beyond the "golden 24-hour period," primary closure is controversial.[93] In these cases, delayed closure is a time-honored practice.[38,71,84] This implies a waiting period of 4 to 5 days before definitive wound closure, during which time the wound is kept open, usually with moist gauze dressings providing drainage, while edema is allowed to subside.[94,95] Antibiotics can be administered to further diminish the risk of infection.[38,87,95]

Other surgeons, however, prefer to proceed with primary repair of late-presenting wounds to achieve a less noticeable scar, although this approach may increase the risk for infection.[16,39,96] This approach has been substantiated by studies suggesting that primary closure of facial human bites can be undertaken with an acceptable risk within 48 hours and even as late as the fourth day after the incident.[40,42,57] However, these studies included mainly low-risk wounds (ie, avulsion type rather than punctures or crush injuries),[97] most of them located on the lips, which are very resistant to the development of infection.

Avulsion bite wounds can pose reconstructive challenges if direct closure is not possible. Attempts to reattach avulsed parts are usually doomed to fail (**Fig. 2**).[35,37,38] In these cases, local skin flaps or composite grafts should be considered, depending on the area involved.[16,18,37,39,41,46,57] Microsurgical replantation has become the standard operation in some centers,[12,98] yet it remains technically demanding.[99] Recently, an extensive soft tissue defect of the face due to a severe dog bite was reconstructed with partial face transplantation.[100]

The presence of overt infection normally precludes suturing the wound. Options include secondary healing with subsequent revision surgery, delayed closure (**Box 2**),[24,38,39] or primary closure with insertion of a drain.[12] Successful immediate primary closure has been reported after debridement with proteolytic agents.[26]

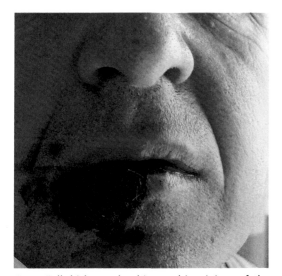

Fig. 2. Full-thickness dog-bite avulsion injury of the lower lip 1 day after an unsuccessful attempt at simple (non-microsurgical) reattachment. Note absence of infection. The defect was later reconstructed with flap surgery. (*Courtesy of* Major Kyriakos Kapagerides, MD.)

ANTIBIOTIC TREATMENT

Antibiotic administration for bite wounds can be either prophylactic or therapeutic.[12,101] In the presence of established infection or any underlying predisposing condition, antibiotic therapy is indicated. However, it remains unclear whether otherwise healthy patients with fresh clinically uninfected wounds benefit from prophylactic antibiotic administration.[18,55,101] Even in these cases, however, antibiotic therapy may actually be therapeutic if enough time has elapsed for bacterial proliferation to reach a level that can result in the development of infection.[11,58,66]

On the basis of figures from a meta-analysis of prophylactic antibiotics for dog-bite wounds,[102] Callaham[67] calculated that as many as 26 patients must be treated with oral antibiotics to prevent 1 infection. Consistently, infection rates in the order of 4% have been reported with primary repair of facial dog-bite wounds without the use of antibiotics.[65,88] On the other hand, with two notable exceptions,[34,46] equally good results have been obtained when antibiotics were administrated.[35,36] Obviously, little evidence supports the value of prophylactic antibiotics in the treatment of dog-bite wounds,[91] although the type of wound, the particular location, and any additional contamination may necessitate antibiotic coverage.[27]

Consensus exists regarding antibiotic prophylaxis for cat-bite wounds because of their high-risk character.[2,12,44,59,70,76,79] Patients with human bites are also serious candidates for antibiotic prophylaxis. Limited evidence suggests that antibiotics for human bites of the face may result in infection rates as low as 2.5%.[37] Furthermore, in a recent study,[38] mainly dealing with high-risk avulsion injuries of the ear, failure to receive at least 48 hours of prophylactic intravenous antibiotics was associated with an increased infection risk following primary closure.

In view of the incomplete debridement permitted on the face,[95] most investigators favor antibiotic prophylaxis for facial bite wounds[12,18,20,35,43,44,46,58,60,81,91] because even low infection rates can seriously compromise cosmetic outcome, especially in children.[77] Furthermore, it has been suggested that primary closure may also increase the risk of infection,[33,92] thus further justifying prophylactic antibiotics in such cases.[56,60,76] Because the indications for antibiotics do not correlate well with the severity of injury,[46] prophylaxis is generally recommended for all bites penetrating the skin.[12,58,77]

For most terrestrial mammal bites, the choice of antibiotics is based on experience with dog, cat, and human bites.[11,50,55,82] Furthermore, because *E corrodens* exhibits similar susceptibility patterns to *Pasteurella* organisms, identical regimens are used for human and most animal bites.[82] Traditional approaches involve selective coverage for the most likely pathogens, including staphylococci, streptococci, and either *Pasteurella* spp for dog and cat bites or *E corrodens*, and oral anaerobes for human bites. Most of these bacteria are susceptible to penicillin, but many strains of *S aureus* and *Prevotella* produce β-lactamase. Thus appropriate regimens should include combinations of penicillin with an antistaphylococcal penicillin or a first-generation cephalosporin,[15,68,70,79] possibly with the addition of metronidazole.

According to current recommendations, amoxicillin/clavulanate is the antimicrobial agent of choice for prophylaxis of bite wounds[27,35,44,59,81,82,91,93,101,103] as it remains active against most animal and human bite-wound isolates.[22,30,49,58,104,105] Few clinical trials have examined the use of amoxicillin/clavulanate in bite cases[66] and reports have appeared noting the failure of amoxicillin/clavulanate in some relevant situations.[92] However, in the series of Kesting and Colleagues,[12] none of the patients who received amoxicillin/clavulanate developed infection, and others have also reported good results with this regimen.[35]

In case of allergy to penicillin, available alternatives include cefuroxime axetil for patients with mild allergy, whereas those with a history of

Table 2
Antimicrobial activity of selected oral agents against common bite-wound pathogens

Agent	Pasteurella Multocida	Staphylococcus Aureus	Streptococcus Spp	Streptococcus "Milleri" (S Anginosus)	Eikenella Corrodens	Prevotella Spp	Fusobacterium Nucleatum
Penicillin	+	−	+	+	+	±	+
Amoxicillin/clavulanate	+	+	+	+	+	+	+
Cefuroxime	+	+	+	+	+	−	−
Doxycycline	+	+	±	−	±	+	+
Erythromycin	−	+	±	±	−	+	−
Azithromycin	+	+	+	+	±	+	±
Ciprofloxacin	+	+	±	0	+	0	0
Moxifloxacin	+	+	+	+	+	+	−
TMP-SMX	+	+	+	+	+	0	0
Clindamycin	0	+	+	+	0	+	+

Key: +, good activity; ±, intermediate activity, probably clinically useful; −, poor activity, clinically unpredictable; 0, no activity.
Abbreviation: TMP-SMX, trimethoprim-sulfamethoxazole.

Data from Goldstein EJC. Outpatient management of dog and cat bite wounds. Fam Pract Recertification 2000;22:67–86; Goldstein EJC, Citron DM, Hudspeth M, et al. In vitro activity of Bay 12–8039, a new 8-methoxyquinolone, compared with the activities of 11 other oral antimicrobial agents against 390 aerobic and anaerobic bacteria isolated from human and animal bite wound skin and soft tissue infections in humans. Antimicrobial Agents Chemother 1997;41:1552–7; and Goldstein EJC, Citron DM, Merriam CV, et al. Comparative in vitro activity of faropenem and 11 other antimicrobial agents against 405 aerobic and anaerobic pathogens isolated from skin and soft tissue infections from animal and human bites. J Antimicrob Chemother 2002;50:411–20.

Table 3
Antimicrobial prophylaxis for common facial bite wounds

Patient	Primary Regimen	Alternative Regimens/Allergy
Adult	Amoxicillin/clavulanate	Clindamycin plus ciprofloxacin Cefuroxime axetil Doxycycline Moxifloxacin Azithromycin
Child	Amoxicillin/clavulanate	Clindamycin plus TMP-SMX Azithromycin
Pregnant	Amoxicillin/clavulanate	Azithromycin

Abbreviation: TMP-SMX, trimethoprim-sulfamethoxazole.

a severe reaction can receive doxycycline[44,81] or a combination of clindamycin with either a fluoroquinolone or trimethoprim-sulfamethoxazole (for children).[56,82,103] Cefuroxime axetil is a recommended alternative for cat-bite wounds,[77,103] but clinical failures have been reported.[106] Moxifloxacin has shown good activity against most bite-wound pathogens, with the exception of most fusobacteria,[58,104,105] and is useful for adult patients allergic to penicillin.[82,106] Azithromycin is probably the most appropriate choice for penicillin-allergic pregnant women or children, for whom tetracyclines, fluoroquinolones, and sulfa compounds are contraindicated.[56,77,82]

For the treatment of established infection, the same basic antibiotic regimens should be followed, except that they should be administered intravenously.[59] Combinations of a β-lactam/β-lactamase inhibitor, such as ampicillin/sulbactam or ticarcillin/clavulanate, moxifloxacin or cefoxitin (because of its anti-anaerobic activity), are all excellent choices;[58,81,103,107] most other second- or third-generation cephalosporins require the addition of an anti-anaerobic agent.[107] The in vitro activity of the previously mentioned agents against most common bite-wound pathogens is listed in **Table 2**, and recommended regimens for prophylaxis are outlined in **Table 3**.

The typical course for antibiotic prophylaxis is 3 to 5 days.[11,55,107] The duration of therapeutic antibiotics varies, depending on the severity of the infection. Most cases of cellulitis require a total of 10 to 14 days.[22,55,56] If cultures were obtained, specific antimicrobial therapy should be based on the culture results.[56] Cases of associated fractures should be treated according to the "therapeutic" rather than the "prophylactic" schedule.

DISCUSSION

Undoubtedly, high-pressure irrigation has a crucial role in the conversion of the contaminated (or even dirty) bite wound into a clean-contaminated environment suitable for subsequent primary closure. Routine use of normal saline is recommended on the premise that emphasis should be placed on the mechanical effect rather than on any antibacterial activity of a more potent solution, which on such a complex wound would be a potential irritant or at best only temporarily effective (see **Box 2**). The use of antiseptic solutions also tends to cause a false sense of security and thus encourages breaching of the treatment protocol. Debridement, if necessary, should not be overzealous. Precise realignment of irregular wound edges is always rewarding in the face and should be preferred to their excision.

Authoritative opinion has pulled back somewhat from previous overconfidence that the vascularity of the face and scalp consistently leads to a favorable outcome for such bite wounds. Realizing that these wounds actually carry a significant risk for infection, influential investigators now recommend antibiotic prophylaxis. This is also the opinion of the author. Two additional factors pertaining to the face can render the management of bite wounds in this area problematic. The first is a substantial risk of occult oral communication with dog-bite injuries of the cheek because of the nature of the dog's occlusion. The second is the presence of the relatively avascular buccal fat pad, which is very developed in children and, once exposed, does not resist infection well. Thus, in cases of deep bites to the cheek, especially in children, after careful exploration and irrigation, antibiotic "prophylaxis" should be started as soon as possible, usually with the first dose administered intravenously.

Determining when to make the repair can be tricky. This is especially true in cases presenting late at night. In such cases, the clinician may prefer a delay to a time when the best expertise is available and operating conditions more suitable. However, delay might make eventual repair more difficult. On the one hand, evidence suggests that some linear lacerations can be safely repaired under antibiotic coverage even when presenting several days after the injury. On the other hand, severely crushed or mangled wounds, besides being at increased risk for infection, tend to become very edematous within hours. Delayed primary closure is indicated in the latter cases to avoid dehiscence because of approximation under tension. Along with experts in the field,[108] the author believes that the decision about timing of repair should be based not so much on the age of the wound as on its appearance.

Finally, as to the proper setting for surgical intervention, most victims with uncomplicated injuries can receive treatment as outpatients. However, even with the most cooperative patients, inadequate assistance or lighting in the crowded emergency department can be very frustrating·and may result in compromise with the principles of facial reconstruction. Therefore, it is preferable to treat even type II injuries in the operating room, if possible, to allow for proper irrigation and meticulous repair of the wound.[109]

SUMMARY

Primary closure is the standard of care for most facial bite wounds, preceded by proper wound irrigation and debridement, where indicated. Administration of antibiotics, preferably on admission, is advisable for all injuries requiring suturing; clean linear lacerations, treated within 3 hours after injury, are possible exceptions. Depending on the clinical appearance of the lesion, patients presenting beyond the first 24 hours should be treated with delayed closure. This option should especially be contemplated for those wounds with gross contamination or with crushed, ischemic, or edematous edges. Serious injuries with bone involvement should be treated according to established protocols. In all cases, clinical judgment should be used and close follow-up is recommended to reduce future complications.

ACKNOWLEDGMENTS

The author wishes to thank Dr. Machi Tarantzopoulou, DDS, for her contribution to the section of antibiotic treatment and for the critical review of the manuscript. The author would also like to thank Professor Michael L. Callaham, MD, for his kind suggestions, and Miss Martha Petromihelaki, for her constant help with the literature search.

REFERENCES

1. Marr JS, Beck AM, Lugo JA. An epidemiologic study of the human bite. Public Health Rep 1979; 94:514–21.
2. Dire DJ. Cat bite wounds: risk factors for infection. Ann Emerg Med 1991;20:973–9.
3. Borud LJ, Friedman DW. Dog bites in New York City. Plast Reconstr Surg 2000;106:989–90.
4. Centers for Disease Control and Prevention. Nonfatal dog-bite related injuries treated in hospital emergency departments—United States, 2001. MMWR Morb Mortal Wkly Rep 2003;52(26):605–10.
5. Schalamon J, Ainoedhofer H, Singer G, et al. Analysis of dog bites in children who are younger than 17 years. Pediatrics 2006;117:374–9.
6. Aghababian RV, Conte JE. Mammalian bite wounds. Ann Emerg Med 1980;9:79–83.
7. Govila A, Rao GS, James JH. Primary reconstruction of a major loss of lower jaw by an animal bite using a "rib sandwich" pectoralis major island flap. Br J Plast Surg 1989;42:101–3.
8. Ogunbodede EO, Arotiba JT. Camel bite injuries of the orofacial region: report of a case. J Oral Maxillofac Surg 1997;55:1174–6.
9. Matter HC, The Sentinel Working Group. The epidemiology of bite and scratch injuries by vertebrate animals in Switzerland. Eur J Epidemiol 1998;14: 483–90.
10. Bahram R, Burke JE, Lanzi GL. Head and neck injury from a leopard attack: case report and review of the literature. J Oral Maxillofac Surg 2004;62:247–9.
11. Freer L. North American wild mammalian injuries. Emerg Med Clin North Am 2004;22:445–73.
12. Kesting MR, Hölzle F, Pox C, et al. Animal bite injuries to the head: 132 cases. Br J Oral Maxillofac Surg 2006;44:235–9.
13. MacBean C, Taylor DMcD, Ashby K. Animal and human bite injuries in Victoria, 1998–2004. Med J Aust 2007;186:38–40.
14. Karlson TA. The incidence of facial injuries from dog bites. JAMA 1984;251:3265–7.
15. Lackmann G-M, Draf W, Isselstein G, et al. Surgical treatment of facial dog bite injuries in children. J Craniomaxillofac Surg 1992;20(2):81–6.
16. Hallock GG. Dog bites of the face with tissue loss. J Craniomaxillofac Trauma 1996;2:49–55.
17. Scheithauer MO, Rettinger G. Bißverletzungen im Kopf-Halsbereich. HNO 1997;45:891–7.
18. Kountakis SE, Chamblee SA, Maillard AAJ, et al. Animal bites to the head and neck. Ear Nose Throat J 1998;77:216–20.
19. Weiss HB, Friedman DI, Coben JH. Incidence of dog bite injuries treated in emergency departments. JAMA 1998;279:51–3.
20. Kahn A, Bauche P, Lamoureux J. Child victims of dog bites treated in emergency departments: a

prospective survey. Eur J Pediatr 2003;162: 254–8.

21. Van Eeckhout GPA, Wylock P. Dog bites: an overview. European Journal of Plastic Surgery 2005;28:233–8.

22. Morgan M, Palmer J. Dog bites. BMJ 2007;334: 413–7.

23. Laskin DM, Donohue WB. Treatment of human bites of the lip. J Oral Surg 1958;16:236–42.

24. Tomasetti BJ, Walker L, Gormley MB, et al. Human bites of the face. J Oral Surg 1979;37:565–8.

25. Ruskin JD, Laney TJ, Wendt SV, et al. Treatment of mammalian bite wounds of the maxillofacial region. J Oral Maxillofac Surg 1993;51:174–6.

26. Baurmash HD, Monto M. Delayed healing human bite wounds of the orofacial area managed with immediate primary closure: treatment rationale. J Oral Maxillofac Surg 2005;63:1391–7.

27. Cunningham LL Jr, Robinson FG, Haug RH, et al. Management of human and animal bites. In: Fonseca RJ, Walker RV, Betts NJ, editors. Oral and maxillofacial trauma. 3rd edition. St Louis (MO): Elsevier Saunders; 2005. p. 843–62.

28. Leach J. Proper handling of sift tissue in the acute phase. Facial Plast Surg 2001;17:227–38.

29. Tu AH, Girotto JA, Singh N, et al. Facial fractures from dog bite injuries. Plast Reconstr Surg 2002; 109:1259–65.

30. Talan DA, Abrahamian FM, Moran GJ, et al. Clinical presentation and bacteriologic analysis of infected human bites in patients presenting to emergency departments. Clin Infect Dis 2003; 37:1481–9.

31. Henry FP, Purcell EM, Eadie PA. The human bite injury: a clinical audit and discussion regarding the management of this alcohol fuelled phenomenon. Emerg Med J 2007;24:455–8.

32. De Munnynck K, Van de Voorde W. Forensic approach of fatal dog attacks: a case report and literature review. Int J Legal Med 2002;116:295–300.

33. Dire DJ, Hogan DE, Riggs MW. A prospective evaluation of risk factors for infections from dog-bite wounds. Acad Emerg Med 1994;1:258–66.

34. Palmer J, Rees M. Dog bites of the face: a 15 year review. Br J Plast Surg 1983;36:315–8.

35. Javaid M, Feldberg L, Gipson M. Primary repair of dog bites to the face: 40 cases. J R Soc Med 1998; 91:414–6 B.

36. Mcheik JN, Vergnes P, Bondonny JM. Treatment of facial dog bite injuries in children: a retrospective study. J Pediatr Surg 2000;35:580–3.

37. Earley MJ, Bardsley AF. Human bites: a review. Br J Plast Surg 1984;37:458–62.

38. Stierman KL, Lloyd KM, De Luca-Pytell D, et al. Treatment and outcome of human bites in the head and neck. Otolaryngol Head Neck Surg 2003;128:795–801.

39. Losken HW, Auchincloss JA. Human bites of the lip. Clin Plast Surg 1984;11:773–5.

40. Venter THJ. Human bites of the face. S Afr Med J 1988;74:277–9.

41. Uchendu BO. Primary closure of human bite losses of the lip. Plast Reconstr Surg 1992;90:841–5.

42. Donkor P, Bankas DO. A study of primary closure of human bite injuries to the face. J Oral Maxillofac Surg 1997;55:479–81.

43. Chidzonga MM. Human bites of the face. S Afr Med J 1998;88:150–2.

44. Goldstein EJC. Outpatient management of dog and cat bite wounds. Family Practice Recertification 2000;22:67–86.

45. Calkins CM, Bensard DD, Partrick DA, et al. Life-threatening dog attacks: a devastating combination of penetrating and blunt injuries. J Pediatr Surg 2001;36:1115–7.

46. Mitchell RB, Nañez G, Wagner JD, et al. Dog bites of the scalp, face, and neck in children. Laryngoscope 2003;113:492–5.

47. Fourie L, Cartilidge D. Fracture of the maxilla following dog bite to the face. Injury 1995;26: 61–2.

48. Goldstein EJC. New horizons in the bacteriology, antimicrobial susceptibility and therapy of animal bite wounds. J Med Microbiol 1998;47:95–7 [editorial].

49. Talan DA, Citron DM, Abrahamian FM, et al. Bacteriologic analysis of infected dog and cat bites. N Engl J Med 1999;340:85–92.

50. Goldstein EJC. Current concepts on animal bites: bacteriology and therapy. Curr Clin Top Infect Dis 1999;19:99–111.

51. Holst E, Rollof J, Larsson L, et al. Characterization and distribution of Pasteurella species recovered from infected humans. J Clin Microbiol 1992;30: 2984–7.

52. Westling K, Farra A, Cars B, et al. Cat bite wound infections: a prospective clinical and microbiological study at three emergency wards in Stockholm, Sweden. J Infect 2006;53:403–7.

53. Brook I. Microbiology of human and animal bite wounds in children. Pediatr Infect Dis J 1987;6: 29–32.

54. Barnham M. Once bitten twice shy: the microbiology of bites. Rev Med Microbiol 1991;2:31–6.

55. Goldstein EJC. Bite wounds and infection. Clin Infect Dis 1992;14:633–40.

56. Abrahamian FM. Dog bites: bacteriology, management, and prevention. Curr Infect Dis Rep 2000;2: 446–53.

57. Agrawal K, Mishra S, Panda KN. Primary reconstruction of major human bite wounds of the face. Plast Reconstr Surg 1992;90:394–8.

58. Brook I. Management of human and animal bite wounds: an overview. Adv Skin Wound Care 2005;18:197–203.

59. Fleisher GR. The management of bite wounds. N Engl J Med 1999;340:138–40 [editorial].

60. Hoff GL, Brawley J, Johnson K. Companion animal issues and the physician. South Med J 1999;92: 651–9.

61. Callaham ML. Treatment of common dog bites: infection risk factors. JACEP 1978;7:83–7.

62. Krizek TJ, Robson MC. Evolution of quantitative bacteriology in wound management. Am J Surg 1975;130:579–84.

63. von Troil-Lindén B, Torkko H, Alaluusua S, et al. Salivary levels of suspected periodontal pathogens in relation to periodontal status and treatment. J Dent Res 1995;74:1789–93.

64. Edlich RF, Spengler MD, Rodeheaver GT, et al. Emergency department management of mammalian bites. Emerg Med Clin North Am 1986;4: 595–604.

65. Maimaris C, Quinton DN. Dog-bite lacerations: a controlled trial of primary wound closure. Arch Emerg Med 1988;5:156–61.

66. Brakenbury PH, Muwanga C. A comparative double blind study of amoxicillin/clavulanate vs placebo in the prevention of infection after animal bites. Arch Emerg Med 1989;6:251–6.

67. Callaham M. Prophylactic antibiotics in dog bite wounds: nipping at the heels of progress. Ann Emerg Med 1994;23:577–9 [editorial].

68. Callaham M. Controversies in antibiotic choices for bite wounds. Ann Emerg Med 1988;17: 1321–30.

69. Callaham ML. Human and animal bites. Top Emerg Med 1982;4:1–13.

70. Weber EJ. Mammalian bites. In: Marx JA, editor. Rosen's emergency medicine: concepts and clinical practice. 6th edition. St Louis (MO): Mosby; 2006. p. 882–92.

71. Lieblich SE, Topazian RG. Infection in the patient with maxillofacial trauma. In: Fonseca RJ, Walker RV, Betts NJ, et al, editors. Oral and maxillofacial trauma. 3rd edition. St Louis (MO): Elsevier Saunders; 2005. p. 1109–30.

72. Capellan O, Hollander JE. Management of lacerations in the emergency department. Emerg Med Clin North Am 2003;21:205–31.

73. Botek AA, Goldberg SH. Management of eyelid dog bites. J Craniomaxillofac Trauma 1996;1: 18–24.

74. Slonim CB. Dog bite-induced canalicular lacerations: a review of 17 cases. Ophthal Plast Reconstr Surg 1996;12:218–22.

75. Abubaker AO. Management of posttraumatic soft tissue infections. Oral Maxillofac Surg Clin North Am 2003;15:139–46.

76. Correira K. Managing dog, cat, and human bite wounds. J Am Acad Physician Assist 2003;16: 28–37.

77. Stefanopoulos PK, Tarantzopoulou AD. Facial bite wounds: management update. Int J Oral Maxillofac Surg 2005;34:464–72.

78. Holm M, Tärnvik A. Hospitalization due to Pasteurella multocida–infected animal bite wounds: correlation with inadequate primary antibiotic medication. Scand J Infect Dis 2000;32:181–3.

79. Dire DJ. Animal bites. In: Singer AJ, Hollander JE, editors. Lacerations and acute wounds: an evidence-based guide. Philadelphia: F.A. Davis; 2003. p. 133–46.

80. Centers for Disease Control and Prevention. Advisory Committee on Immunization Practices. Preventing tetanus, diphtheria, and pertussis among adults: use of tetanus toxoid, reduced diphtheria toxoid and acellular pertussis vaccine. MMWR Recomm Rep 2006;55(RR17):1–37.

81. Bartlett JG. Johns Hopkins antibiotic guide: bite wounds. Available at: http://prod.hopkins-abxguide. org/diagnosis/soft_tissue/bite_wounds.

82. Moran GJ, Talan DA, Abrahamian FM. Antimicrobial prophylaxis for wounds and procedures in the emergency department. Infect Dis Clin North Am 2008;22:117–43.

83. Chisholm CD. Wound evaluation and cleansing. Emerg Med Clin North Am 1992;10:665–72.

84. Simon B, Hern HG Jr. Wound management principles. In: Marx JA, editor. Rosen's emergency medicine: concepts and clinical practice. 6th edition. Philadelphia: Mosby Elsevier; 2006. p. 842–57.

85. Callaham M. Prophylactic antibiotics in common dog bite wounds: a controlled study. Ann Emerg Med 1980;9:410–4.

86. Hollander JE, Singer AJ. Laceration management. Ann Emerg Med 1999;34:356–67.

87. Brancato JC. Minor wound preparation and irrigation. Up to date; version 16.1. Available at: www. uptodate.com.

88. Guy RJ, Zook EG. Successful treatment of acute head and neck dog bite wounds without antibiotics. Ann Plast Surg 1986;17:45–8.

89. Dire DJ, Welsh AP. A comparison of wound irrigation solutions used in the emergency department. Ann Emerg Med 1990;19:704–8.

90. Fernandez R, Griffiths R, Ussia C. Effectiveness of solutions, techniques and pressure in wound cleansing. The Joanna Briggs Institute Reports 2004;2:231–70.

91. Chaudhry MA, MacNamara AF, Clark S. Is the management of dog bite wounds evidence based? A postal survey and review of the literature. Eur J Emerg Med 2004;11:313–7.

92. Chen E, Hornig S, Shepherd SM, et al. Primary closure of mammalian bites. Acad Emerg Med 2000;7:157–61.

93. Vasconez HC. Soft tissue injuries. In: Goldwyn RM, Cohen MN, editors. The unfavorable result in

plastic surgery: avoidance and treatment. 3rd edition. Philadelphia: Lippincott Williams & Wilkins; 2001. p. 453–65.

94. Dimick AR. Delayed wound closure: indications and techniques. Ann Emerg Med 1988;17:1303–4.

95. Dufresne CR, Manson PN. Pediatric facial injuries. In: Mathes SJ, editor. Plastic surgery. 2nd edition. Philadelphia: Saunders Elsevier; 2006. p. 381–462.

96. Eppley BL, Bhuller A. Principles of facial soft tissue injury repair. In: Ward Booth P, Eppley BL, Schmelzeisen R, editors. Maxillofacial trauma and esthetic facial reconstruction. Edinburgh: Churchill Livingstone; 2003. p. 107–20.

97. Ruskin JD. Discussion: a study of primary closure of human bite injuries to the face. J Oral Maxillofac Surg 1997;55:481–2.

98. Hussain G, Thomson S, Zielinski V. Nasal amputation due to human bite: microsurgical replantation. Aust N Z J Surg 1997;67:382–4.

99. Flores RL, Hazen A, Galiano RD, et al. Non-extremity replantation: the management of amputations of the facial parts and testicle. Clin Plast Surg 2007;34:197–210.

100. Devauchelle B, Badet L, Lengelé B, et al. First human face allograft: early report. Lancet 2006;368:203–9.

101. Nakamura Y, Daya M. Use of appropriate antimicrobials in wound management. Emerg Med Clin North Am 2007;25:159–76.

102. Cummings P. Antibiotics to prevent infection in patients with dog bite wounds: a meta-analysis of randomized trials. Ann Emerg Med 1994;23:535–40.

103. Gilbert DN, Moellering RC Jr, Eliopoulos GM, et al. The Sanford guide to antimicrobial therapy 2007.

37th edition. Sperryville (VA): Antimicrobial Therapy, Inc; 2007. p. 46–7.

104. Goldstein EJC, Citron DM, Hudspeth M, et al. In vitro activity of Bay 12–8039, a new 8-methoxyquinolone, compared to the activities of 11 other oral antimicrobial agents against 390 aerobic and anaerobic bacteria isolated from human and animal bite wound skin and soft tissue infections in humans. Antimicrobial Agents Chemother 1997;41:1552–7.

105. Goldstein EJC, Citron DM, Merriam CV, et al. Comparative in vitro activity of faropenem and 11 other antimicrobial agents against 405 aerobic and anaerobic pathogens isolated from skin and soft tissue infections from animal and human bites. J Antimicrob Chemother 2002;50:411–20.

106. Draenert R, Kunzelmann M, Roggenkamp A, et al. Infected cat-bite wound treated successfully with moxifloxacin after failure of parenteral cefuroxime and ciprofloxacin. Eur J Clin Microbiol Infect Dis 2005;24:288–90.

107. Stevens DL, Bisno AL, Chambers HF, et al. Practice guidelines for the diagnosis and management of skin and soft-tissue infections. Clin Infect Dis 2005;41:1373–406.

108. Cohen MN. Soft tissue injuries. In: Goldwyn RM, Cohen MN, editors. The unfavorable result in plastic surgery: avoidance and treatment. 3rd edition. Philadelphia: Lippincott Williams & Wilkins; 2001. p. 465–8 [discussion].

109. Henderson JM. Comment on ref. 77. In: McIntyre FM, editor. Year book of dentistry 2006. Philadelphia: Elsevier Mosby; 2006. p. 173.

Use of Prophylactic Antibiotics in Preventing Infection of Traumatic Injuries

A. Omar Abubaker, DMD, PhD

KEYWORDS

• Prophylactic• Soft tissue • Infection • Trauma

Approximately 11.8 million wounds were treated in the emergency departments in the United States in 2005.[1] At least 7.3 million lacerations are treated annually[2] and an additional 2 million outpatient visits each year occur for treatment of wounds caused by cutting or piercing objects.[3] Half of these traumatic wounds are located on the head and neck,[3,4] This makes it important for clinicians to understand how best to prevent infections following traumatic soft tissue injuries, as well as traumatic bony injuries, in these areas.

The primary goal in the management of traumatic wounds is to achieve rapid healing with optimal functional and esthetic results.[5] This is best accomplished by providing an environment that prevents infection of the wound during healing. Such care includes adequate overall medical assessment of the patient; proper wound evaluation and preparation; adequate anesthesia and hemostasis; reduction of tissue contamination by wound cleansing, debridement of devitalized tissue, and removal of any foreign bodies; and correct wound closure. Several reviews describe the principles and details of this phase of wound care.[6]

Despite good wound care, some infections still occur. Accordingly, some investigators argue that prophylactic antibiotics have an important role in the management of certain types of wounds.[7] This article reviews the basis of antibiotic use in preventing wound infection in general and its use in oral and facial wounds in particular. See the article by Stefanopoulos elsewhere in this issue for a discussion of the role of antibiotics in the management of bite wounds.

PROPHYLACTIC ANTIBIOTICS IN PATIENTS WITH SKIN WOUNDS

The term *prophylactic antibiotics* implies the use of such antibiotics as a preventive measure in the absence of an established infection.[8,9] Although virtually all traumatic wounds can be considered contaminated with bacteria to some extent, only a small percentage eventually become infected. Accordingly, it is possible that only a subset of high-risk wounds or patients stand to benefit from prophylactic antibiotics.[7] Estimates of the incidence of traumatic wound infection vary widely, depending on the method of study and the population examined, but most studies have found an incidence of 4.5% to 6.3%.[10–13] In a meta-analysis of seven studies, the wound infection rates in the control populations ranged from 1.1% to 12% with a mean of 6%.[14]

When considering the role of antibiotics in preventing wound infection, it is important to consider the risk factors for infection. These factors relate to the nature of the host, the characteristics of the wound, and the treatment used.[15] The host risk factors include extreme young or old age; medical problems, such as diabetes mellitus, chronic renal failure, obesity, malnutrition, and immunocompromising illnesses; and such therapies as corticosteroids and chemotherapeutic agents.[8,9,16,17] Wound factors that increase risk include high

Department of Oral and Maxillofacial Surgery, School of Dentistry, Virginia Commonwealth University, Virginia Commonwealth University Medical Center, 521 North 11th Street, PO Box 980566, Richmond, VA 23298, USA.
E-mail address: abubaker@vcu.edu

Oral Maxillofacial Surg Clin N Am 21 (2009) 259–264
doi:10.1016/j.coms.2008.12.001
1042-3699/08/$ – see front matter © 2009 Elsevier Inc. All rights reserved.

bacterial counts in the wound; oil contamination; and crush injury. Risk of infection also varies according to wound depth, configuration, and size.[7,18] Wounds associated with tendons, joints, and bones; puncture wounds; intraoral wounds; and most mammalian wounds are also considered at high risk for infection. Certain treatments, such as the use of epinephrine-containing solutions, may also increase the risk of infection. Furthermore, risk of infection increases with the number of sutures. Finally, risk of infection may be higher with an inexperienced treating doctor than with an experienced one.[19]

When antibiotics are used to prevent infections in traumatic wounds, certain indications are often cited. Such indications include wounds associated with open joints or fractures, human or animal bites, and intraoral lacerations. Despite limited evidence, antibiotics also are recommended for heavily contaminated wounds (eg, those involving soil, feces, saliva, vaginal secretions, or other contaminants).[20] Prophylactic antibiotics also are advocated for traumatic wounds in patients who have prosthetic devices and for preventing bacteremia in patients at risk for developing endocarditis.[20,21] Systemic antibiotics also are recommended when there is a lapse of more than 3 hours since injury, when there is lymphedematous tissue involvement, and when the host is immunocompromised.[22,23]

According to the principles of presurgical prophylaxis, antibiotics, if they are to be given at all, should be administered as soon as possible after the injury, if possible within the first 3 hours, and continued for 3 to 5 days.[7,22,24] The antibiotic therapy should also be directed against the most common skin pathogens, *Staphylococcus aureus* and streptococci.[22] Cloxacillin and first-generation cephalosporins are appropriate as first-line therapy.

Despite the frequent use of prophylactic antibiotics to prevent traumatic wound infections, some clinicians still have reservations about the effectiveness of their use. Some investigators argue that most uncomplicated wounds heal without systemic antibiotic therapy.[22] In addition, in many situations, prophylactic antibiotics not only fail to reduce the overall rate of infection, but also may skew the bacteriology toward more unusual or resistant pathogens.[7] In fact, clinical studies fail to demonstrate a lower infection rate among patients with uncomplicated wounds treated with prophylactic antibiotics than among control subjects,[25] and no randomized trials have shown a clear benefit of antibiotic prophylaxis for simple wounds in immunocompetent patients.[25-30] Furthermore, a meta-analysis of randomized trials found no

benefit from the use of prophylactic antibiotics for simple wounds.[24]

Several randomized, controlled studies have examined the ability of antibiotics to prevent infection of simple nonbite wounds managed in the emergency department. A meta-analysis of seven of these studies showed that wound infection rates in the control populations ranged from 1.1% to 12%, with a mean of 6%, with patients treated with antibiotics having a slightly greater risk of infection than untreated controls.[14] More detailed analysis of several subgroups looked at whether or not the wounds were sutured, whether the wounds were located on the hands or elsewhere, what was the route of antibiotic administration (oral versus intramuscular), and what antibiotic type was employed. This analysis also failed to show any benefit for the use of systemic prophylactic antibiotics. In 1995, Cummings and Del Becaro[14] concluded that there was little justification for the routine administration of antibiotics to patients who had simple nonbite wounds managed in the emergency department. However, these investigators were unable to examine the potential benefits of antibiotics in high-risk groups because most of these were excluded from their clinical trials. Accordingly, selection bias remains a problematic issue, with most of the published studies looking at the role of antibiotics in management of traumatic wounds in the emergency department.[15,20]

USE OF PROPHYLACTIC ANTIBIOTICS FOR PREVENTION OF INFECTION OF INTRAORAL WOUNDS

Intraoral wounds, including tongue lacerations and orocutaneous wounds, are commonly encountered in the emergency department. Such wounds can involve the mucosa only or the mucosa and adjacent skin, so-called "through-and-through" lacerations. These wounds are often the result of penetration of the lips by the patient's teeth following minor or major trauma or seizures. Most emergency medicine textbooks consider larger mucosal wounds, particularly those that are through-and-through wounds, to be dirty wounds and at high risk for infection because of the oral bacterial flora. These books generally recommend a course of prophylactic antibiotics to prevent infection after these wounds are repaired.[31,32] Infection has been reported in up to 12% of wounds involving the mucosa only and in up to 33% of through-and-through lacerations[33] Altieri and colleagues[34] studied the benefits of 3 days of penicillin prophylaxis in a randomized, controlled trial of 100 intraoral lacerations managed in a pediatric emergency department. The overall infection rate was found to be 6.4%, with no statistically significant difference between the control (8.5%) and the penicillin (4.4%) groups. Although this study had a limited number of patients enrolled, it concluded that routine antibiotic prophylaxis is unwarranted for simple intraoral lacerations in children, although it may be beneficial in sutured wounds.[35] Steel and colleagues[33] conducted a prospective, randomized, double-blind, controlled study of 5 days of oral penicillin versus placebo therapy in adults. They found a statistically significant difference in the infection rates between compliant patients in the two groups (6.7% for penicillin versus 18.8% in the placebo group). In a subgroup of those patients who had through-and-through lacerations, 7% of the treatment group versus 27% of the control group developed wound infections. These investigators could not conclusively recommend prophylactic penicillin for adults with intraoral lacerations treated within 24 hours after injury. However, the investigators felt that noncompliant patients and those who had through-and-through lacerations may benefit from a course of prophylactic penicillin.[33] Penicillin-allergic patients should receive clindamycin.[15]

Mark and Granquist[35] reviewed the literature on the use of prophylactic oral antibiotics for treatment of intraoral wounds. Only four clinical research articles fulfilled their criteria for inclusion in the review.[33,34,36,37] They concluded that prophylactic oral antibiotics play an inconclusive role in the treatment of intraoral wounds. They also concluded that all published randomized studies to date have failed to demonstrate a statistically significant difference in wound infection rates when antibiotics are compared with placebo or routine wound care. The only placebo-controlled, double-blind, randomized clinical trial evaluating the efficacy of oral prophylactic antibiotic use in simple intraoral wounds had small enrollment numbers and accordingly failed to conclusively demonstrate a statistically significant benefit of such use. Mark and Granquist[35] recommended that until a larger clinical trial is performed, treatment decisions on the use of prophylactic antibiotics for intraoral wounds should be guided by clinical judgment of the practitioner.

The value of antibiotic prophylaxis for lacerations of the tongue is less well studied, although one underpowered study reported no infections in 28 children managed without antibiotics.[38] Accordingly, there is insufficient evidence to make any definitive recommendations with regard to antibiotic prophylaxis for tongue or intraoral lacerations in children.[21]

TOPICAL ANTIBIOTICS FOR TREATMENT OF TRAUMATIC WOUNDS

Application of topical antibiotic ointments has often been proposed to help reduce infection rates and prevent scab formation.[22,25,30,39] Ointments containing bacitracin, neomycin, or polymyxin have been routinely used on simple lacerations by many emergency physicians in the United States.[40] Animal studies have shown that topical antimicrobials inside the wound before closure may reduce the infection rate in contaminated wounds.[41] One double-blind, randomized human trial found a 5% infection rate with antibiotic ointment compared with an unexpectedly high 17.6% rate with a petrolatum jelly control.[42] Other studies, however, have found no significant reduction in infection rates with topical antibiotics.[43] Because of the higher risk of infection with crush injuries when compared with sharp lacerations, some experts recommend topical antibiotics only for stellate wounds with abraded skin edges,[44] but this is not based on comparative trial data. So far, the effectiveness of topical antibiotic ointments in managing minor wounds has not been properly investigated.[7,21] Moreover, despite the frequent use of topical antibiotics, surprisingly few studies have assessed their efficacy after suture wound closure.[7]

ANTIBIOTIC PROPHYLAXIS IN PATIENTS WITH OPEN FRACTURES AND JOINT WOUNDS

Open fracture and joint wounds are a recognizable risk for microbial contamination and subsequent development of osteomyelitis. Any break in the skin (or mucosa) over a fracture that could allow for bacterial access to bone should be considered an open fracture. Open fractures and joint wounds are often classified into three categories according to the mechanism of injury, severity of soft tissue damage, configuration of the fracture, and degree of contamination.[45,46] Type I is an open fracture with a skin wound that is clean and less than 1 cm long; type II is an open fracture with a laceration that is more than 1 cm long, but without evidence of extensive soft tissue damage, flaps, or avulsion; and type III is either an open segmental fracture or an open fracture with extensive soft tissue damage or a traumatic amputation. A prospective, randomized, controlled trial by Patzakis and colleagues[47] on the importance of antibiotics in the treatment of open fractures showed that the infection rates were 13.9%, 10%, and 2.3% in the placebo, penicillin, and cephalosporin groups, respectively. In a follow-up study, Patzakis and Wilkins[48] showed that the single most important factor in reducing the infection rate was early (<3 hours) administration of antibiotics that provide antibacterial activity against both gram-positive and gram-negative organisms.[48] A Cochrane Database review concluded that antibiotics reduce the incidence of infection in open fractures of the limbs when compared with no antibiotics or placebo.[49]

Most investigators agree that the use of antibiotics in the management of open fractures and joint wounds is appropriate. However, the duration of therapy and the optimal antibiotic choices remain unresolved issues.[8] Current recommendations with regard to duration are to continue treatment for 24 hours after wound closure in type I and II injuries and for 72 hours, or for 24 hours after wound closure, in type III injuries.[45,50] For type I and II open fractures, *S aureus*, streptococci spp, and aerobic gram-negative bacilli are the most common infecting organisms, and the antibiotic of choice is a first- or second-generation cephalosporin.[45,51] An extended-spectrum quinolone (eg, gatifloxacin or moxifloxacin) is an alternative antibiotic regimen that is currently the preferred choice in the military.[52,53] Type III open fractures may require better coverage for gram-negative organisms by the addition of an aminoglycoside to a cephalosporin.[45] For severe injures with soil or fecal contamination and tissue damage with areas of ischemia, it is recommended that penicillin be added to provide coverage against anaerobes, particularly Clostridia spp.[8] Antibiotic coverage for other bacteria may also be needed for certain environmental exposures, such as farm accidents (*Clostridium*), combat casualty wounds (*Acinetobacter, Pseudomonas, Clostridium*), fresh water exposure (*Aeromonas, Pseudomonas*), and salt water exposure (*Aeromonas, Vibrio*).[51,54]

Antibiotic therapy for prophylactic management of open fractures resulting from gunshot wounds warrants special consideration and depends in part on whether the injury was caused by a low- or high-velocity missile.[8] In fractures associated with low-velocity wounds treated with a closed technique, the infection rate with antibiotic prophylaxis is about the same as the infection rate without antibiotic prophylaxis (3% in both groups).[55] However, wounds caused by high-velocity gunshot injuries are associated with increased risk of infection, and antibiotic therapy is generally recommended for 48 to 72 hours.[56] Although a first-generation cephalosporin with or without an aminoglycoside is recommended for most patients, penicillin should be added to provide additional anaerobic coverage of Clostridia spp in grossly contaminated wounds.[57] The Eastern Surgical Society for the Surgery of Trauma

has developed treatment guidelines for use of prophylactic antibiotics in open fractures. For type I and type II fractures, these guidelines recommend antibiotic therapy directed against gram-positive bacteria (first-generation cephalosporins) be administered within 6 hours of the injury and for 24 hours after wound closure. For type III fractures, antibiotic therapy should be directed against gram-positive and gram-negative bacteria, be given within 6 hours following the fracture, and be continued for 72 hours, or for 24 hours after wound closure.[45]

In the oral and maxillofacial region, guidelines in the literature are less clear-cut about the use of prophylactic antibiotic to prevent infection when soft tissue injury is associated with facial fractures. A systematic review revealed four randomized studies that examined the possible benefit of prophylactic antibiotics in such situations.[58] This review included studies related to facial factures with and without facial skin or mucosal lacerations.[59–63] The investigators concluded that only compound fractures of the body and angle of the mandible would benefit from a short-term course of prophylactic antibiotics (<48 hours). The review did not address the relationship between soft tissue lacerations, facial fractures, and the use of prophylactic antibiotics, although the investigators suggested that the benefit of prophylactic antibiotics is likely to be related to their effect on bacterial contamination from the dentition and through the periodontal ligament.[58]

SUMMARY

The wide use, misuse, and overuse of prophylactic antibiotics likely contribute significantly to overall health care cost. One of the areas of potential misuse of these agents is in the prevention of infection of traumatic wounds. This review shows that despite the widespread use of prophylactic antibiotics to prevent infection of wound injuries, the scientific data to support such wide use are limited to specific situations and for limited periods of time. These situations include those involving immunocompromised patients; grossly contaminated wounds; delayed wound closure; patients at high risk for endocarditis; patients with open fractures and joint wounds; and high-velocity gunshot wounds. There may also be a benefit of such use for short duration when facial or oral lacerations are associated with compound fractures of the mandible and in through-and-through lacerations of the mouth in adults. There appears to be no benefit for prophylactic antibiotics for simple facial skin lacerations, tongue lacerations, and intraoral lacerations when they are not associated with facial fractures.

REFERENCES

1. Nawar EW, Niska RW, Xu J. National Hospital Ambulatory Medical Care Survey: 2005 emergency department summary. Advance data from vital health statistics. No. 386. Hyattsville (MD): National Center for Health Statistics; 2007.
2. Singer AJ, Thode HC, Hollander JE. National trends in ED lacerations between 1992 and 2002. Am J Emerg Med 2006;24:183–8.
3. Hing E, Cherry DK, Woodwell DA. National Ambulatory Medical Care Survey: 2004 summary. Advance data from vital and health statistics. No. 374. Hyattsville (MD): National Center for Health Statistics; 2006.
4. Hollander GE, Singer JA. State of the art laceration management. Ann Emerg Med 1999;34:356–67.
5. Singer AJ, Dagum AB. Current management of acute cutaneous wounds. N Engl J Med 2008;359:1037–46.
6. Capellan O, Hollander JE. Management of lacerations in the emergency department. Emerg Med Clin North Am 2003;21:205–31.
7. Moran GJ, Talan DA, Abrahamian FD. Antimicrobial prophylaxis for wounds and procedures in the emergency department. Infect Dis Clin North Am 2008; 22:117–43.
8. Holtom PD. Antibiotic prophylaxis: current recommendations. J Am Acad Orthop Surg 2006;14: S98–100.
9. Mangram AJ, Horan TC, Pearson ML, et al. Guideline for prevention of surgical site infection. 1999; Hospital Infection Control Practices Advisory Committee. Infect Control Hosp Epidemiol 1999;20:250–78.
10. Gosnold JK. Infection rate of sutured wounds. Practitioner 1977;218:584–5.
11. Hutton PA, Jones BM, Law DJ. Depot penicillin as prophylaxis in accidental wounds. Br J Surg 1978; 65:549–50.
12. Rutherford WH, Spence R. Infection in wounds sutured in the accident and emergency department. Ann Emerg Med 1980;9:350–2.
13. Thirlby RC, Blair AJ, Thal ER. The value of prophylactic antibiotics for simple lacerations. Surg Gynecol Obstet 1983;156:212–6.
14. Cummings P, Del Beccaro MA. Antibiotics to prevent infection of simple wounds: a meta-analysis of randomized studies. Am J Emerg Med 1995;13:396–400.
15. Nakamura Y, Daya M. Use of appropriate antimicrobials in wound management. Emerg Med Clin North Am 2007;25:159–76.
16. Singer AJ, Hollander JE, Quinn JV. Evaluation and management of traumatic lacerations. N Engl J Med 1997;337:1142–8.
17. Cruse PJE, Foord R. A five-year prospective study of 23,469 surgical wounds. Arch Surg 1973;107:206–9.
18. Hollander JE, Singer AJ, Valantine SM, et al. Risk infection in patients with traumatic laceration. Acad Emerg Med 2001;8:716–20.
19. Lammers RL, Hudson DL, Seaman ME. Prediction of traumatic wound infection with a neural network-derived decision model. Am J Emerg Med 2003; 21:1–7.
20. Wedmore IS. Wound care: modern evidence in the treatment of man's age-old injuries. Emerg Med Pract 2005;7:1–24.
21. Goulin S, Patel H. Office management of minor wounds. Can Fam Physician 2001;47:769–74.
22. Eron LJ. Targeting lurking pathogens in acute traumatic and chronic wounds. J Emerg Med 1999;17: 189–95.
23. Horetg FM, King C. Textbook of pediatric emergency procedures. Baltimore (MD): Williams & Wilkins; 1997. Chap 7, p. 43–9; Chap1101, p. 125–39.
24. Gravett A, Sterner S, Clinton JE, et al. A trial of povidone-iodine in the prevention of infection in sutured lacerations. Ann Emerg Med 1987;16:167–71.
25. Barkin RM, Caputo GL, Jaffe DM, et al. Pediatric emergency medicine, concepts and clinical practice. 2nd edition. St. Louis (MO): Mosby; 1997. Chap 32, p. 439–75.
26. Quinn JV, Wells G, Sutcliffe T, et al. Tissue adhesive versus suture wound repair at 1 year: randomized clinical trial correlating early, 3-month, and 1-year cosmetic outcome. Ann Emerg Med 1998;32:645–9.
27. Singer AJ, Hollander JB, Valantine SM, et al. Prospective, randomized, controlled trials of tissue adhesive 2-octycyanoacrylate vs standard wound closure techniques for laceration repair. Acad Emerg Med 1998;5:94–9.
28. Bruns TB, Simon Hk, McLario DJ, et al. Laceration repair using a tissue adhesive in a children's emergency department. Pediatrics 1996;98:673–5.
29. Quinn JV, Drzewiecki A, Li MM, et al. A randomized, controlled trial comparing a tissue adhesive with suturing in the repair of pediatric facial lacerations. Ann Emerg Med 1993;22:23–7.
30. Kunisad T, Yamada K, Oda S, et al. Investigation on the efficacy of povidone-iodine against antiseptic-resistant species. Dermatology 1997;195(Suppl 2): 14–8.
31. Tintinalli JE, Kelen GD, Stapczynski JS, editors. Emergency medicine: a comprehensive study guide. 6th edition. New York: McGraw-Hill; 2004.
32. Marx JA, Hockberger RS, Walls RM, editors. Marx: Rosen's emergency medicine: concepts and clinical practice. 6th edition. Philadelphia: Mosby Elsevier; 2006.
33. Steel MT, Sainsbury CR, Robinson WA, et al. Prophylactic penicillin for intraoral wounds. Ann Emerg Med 1989;18:847–52.
34. Altieri M, Brasch L, Getson P. Antibiotic prophylaxis in intraoral wounds. Am J Emerg Med 1986;4:507–10.

35. Mark DJ, Granquist EJ. Are prophylactic oral antibiotics indicated for the treatment of intraoral wounds? Ann Emerg Med 2008;52:368–72.

36. Goldberg MH. Antibiotics and oral and oral-cutaneous lacerations. J Oral Surg 1965;23:117–22.

37. Paterson JA, Cardo VA Jr, Stratigos GT. An examination of antibiotic prophylaxis in oral and maxillofacial surgery. J Oral Surg 1970;28:753–9.

38. Lamell CW, Fraone G, Casamassimo MS, et al. Presenting characteristics and treatment outcomes for tongue lacerations in children. Pediatr Dent 1999;21:34–8.

39. Bikowski J. Secondarily infected wounds and dermatoses: a diagnosis and treatment guide. J Emerg Med 1999;17:197–206.

40. Howell JM, Chisholm CD. Outpatient wound preparation and care: a national survey. Ann Emerg Med 1992;24:976–81.

41. Edlich RF, Smith QT, Edgerton MT. Resistance of the surgical wound to antimicrobial prophylaxis and its mechanisms of development. Am J Surg 1973;126: 583–91.

42. Dire DJ, Coppola M, Dwyer DA, et al. A prospective evaluation of topical antibiotics for preventing infections in uncomplicated soft-tissue wounds repaired in the ED. Acad Emerg Med 1995;2:4–10.

43. Caro D, Reynolds KW. An investigation to evaluate a topical antibiotic in the prevention of wound sepsis in a casualty department. Br J Clin Pract 1967;21:605–7.

44. Edlich RF, Sutton ST. Post repair wound care revisited. Acad Emerg Med 1995;2:2–3.

45. Luchette FA, Bone LB, Born CT, et al. East Practice Management Guidelines Work Group: practice management guidelines for prophylactic antibiotic use in open fractures. Available at: http://www.east. org/. Accessed November 18, 2006.

46. Gustilo RB, Mendoza RM, Williams DN. Problems in the management of type III (severe) open fractures. A new classification of type III open fractures. J Trauma 1984;24:742–6.

47. Patzakis MJ, Harvey JP Jr, Ivler D. The role of antibiotics in the management of open fractures. J Bone Joint Surg Am 1974;56:532–41.

48. Patzakis MJ, Wilkins J. Factors influencing infection rate in open fracture wounds. Clin Orthop Relat Res 1989;243:36–40.

49. Gosselin RI, Roberts I, Gillespie WJ. Antibiotics for preventing infection in open limb fractures. Cochrane Database Syst Rev 2004;(1):CD003764.

50. Calhoun J, Sexton DJ, et al. Adult posttraumatic osteomyelitis. Up to Date 2006; ver 14.3. Available at: www. uptodate.com. Acccessed November 16, 2008.

51. Templeman DC, Gulli B, Tsukayama DT, et al. Update on the management of open fractures of the tibial shaft. Clin Orthop Relat Res 1998;350:18–25.

52. Patzakis MJ, Banis RS, Lee J, et al. Prospective randomized, double-blind study comparing agent antibiotic therapy, ciprofloxacin, to combination antibiotic therapy in open fracture wounds. J Orthop Trauma 2000;14:529–33.

53. Butler F. Antibiotics in facial combat casualty care 2002. Mil Med 2003;168:911–4.

54. Davis SC, Cazzaniga AL, Eaglstein WH, et al. Over-the-counter topical antimicrobials: effective treatments? Arch Dermatol Res 2005;297:190–5.

55. Dickey RL, Barnes BC, Kearns RJ, et al. Efficacy of antibiotics in low-velocity gunshot fractures. J Orthop Trauma 1989;3:6–10.

56. Heenessy MJ, Banks HH, Leach RB. Extremity gunshot wound and gunshot fracture in civilian practice. Clin Orthop Relat Res 1976;114:296–303.

57. Simpson BM, Wilson RH, Grant RE. Antibiotic therapy in gunshot wound injuries. Clin Orthop Relat Res 2003;408:82–5.

58. Anderasen JO, Jensen S, Schwartz O, et al. A systemic review of prophylactic antibiotics in the surgical treatment of maxillofacial fractures. J Oral Maxillofac Surg 2006;64:1664–8.

59. Chole RA, Yee J. Antibiotic prophylaxis for facial fractures. Arch Otolaryngol Head Neck Surg 1987; 113:1055–7.

60. Zallen RD, Curry JT. A study of antibiotic usage in compound mandibular fractures. J Oral Surg 1975; 33:431–4.

61. Aderhold L, Jung H, Frenkel G. Untersuchungen über den wert einer Antibiotika Prophylaxe bei kiefer-Gesichtsverletzungen-eine prospective studie. Dtsch Zahnärztl Z 1983;38:402–7.

62. Gerlach KL, Pape HD. Untersuchungen zur Antibiotikaprophylaxe bei der operativen Behandlung von Unterkieferfrakturen. Dtsch Z Mund Kiefer Gesichtschir 1988;12:497–502.

63. Abubaker AO, Rollert MK. Postoperative antibiotic prophylaxis in mandibular fractures: a preliminary randomized, double-blind, and placebo-controlled clinical study. J Oral Maxillofac Surg 2001;59: 1415–9.

Index

Note: Page numbers of article titles are in **boldface** type.

Oral Maxillofacial Surg Clin N Am 21 (2009) 265–268
doi:10.1016/S1042-3699(09)00034-X
1042-3699/09/$ – see front matter © 2009 Elsevier Inc. All rights reserved.

Moving?

Make sure your subscription moves with you!

To notify us of your new address, find your **Clinics Account Number** (located on your mailing label above your name), and contact customer service at:

E-mail: elspcs@elsevier.com

800-654-2452 (subscribers in the U.S. & Canada)
314-453-7041 (subscribers outside of the U.S. & Canada)

Fax number: 314-523-5170

Elsevier Periodicals Customer Service
11830 Westline Industrial Drive
St. Louis, MO 63146

*To ensure uninterrupted delivery of your subscription, please notify us at least 4 weeks in advance of move.

ELSEVIER

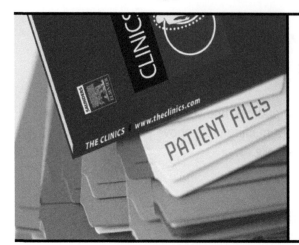
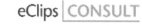
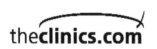

Printed and bound by CPI Group (UK) Ltd, Croydon, CR0 4YY

03/10/2024

01040362-0008